SOMATIC TRAUMA HEALING

The at-home DIY crash course in experiencing true body awareness through somatic secrets anyone can do & insider techniques your therapist doesn't want you to know about

ASCENDING VIBRATIONS

Ascending Vibrations

CONTENTS

BONUS GUIDED MEDITATION

Wouldn't it be nice to have even more motivation, inspiration, and courage on your spiritual path? As a sincere "Thank you" for reading this book, you can claim your downloadable 10 minute Energy Healing guided meditation Mp3 below.

Do you want to release toxicity within & realign with your true energy?

- STAND FIRM, say no, & set boundaries by owning your unique power & energy
- Become a magnet for other high vibrational energies
- Protect yourself from those in your life who have energy imbalances & are lowering your vibration

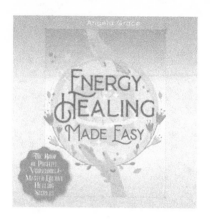

Go to this link to Get Your Free 10 minute Energy Healing Guided Meditation Mp3:

bit.ly/energyhealingfree

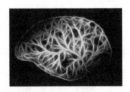

INTRODUCTION

It is a given that many of the books on Somatic Healing Therapy aim to help the reader with their myriad issues directly. However, the complex scientific terminology & hard-to-follow exercises commonplace in such titles can often result in a perplexed reader left scratching their head. This book is different. This book is self-help in the truest sense of the word. Nothing in here is going to be complicated or bewildering. Everything I write is going to be easy for you to understand and easy to follow. If there are more challenging concepts contained within the chapters, then I will break them down to the point where anyone new to somatic healing will be able to understand. You won't need a doctor or a wall of scientific degrees to work out what the author is trying to convey. This book is for anybody and everybody.

The exercises contained in this book are not going to be so difficult that you need to go and get help from your neighbors or consult a professional Somatic Therapist to help you. No, these will be simple exercises that anybody, no matter how young or old, can easily follow and carry out in the safety of their home.

I appreciate that if you are interested in this book, it may well mean that you have been through some very stressful or traumatic experiences and are searching for healing. Please remember I am here to support you and encourage you through this journey. I will avoid using particular language and mentioning specific situations that could trigger a recurrence of that trauma in you. This book is a safe haven for you. You should always be able to find that peace and comfort whenever you are dipping into this book. It should be your guide when you need to practice exercises to help with your healing journey. These are not exercises to use just once and never bother with again. They are exercises that you can use daily to encourage the healing within you. Don't worry: You don't need to prescribe to some mystical religion or follow a shamanic leader to take part in recovery. Everything here is pragmatic and for your enjoyment, knowledge, and enlightenment. It does not require you to change your whole belief system to benefit from it.

I will also be discussing trauma and how it impacts and affects all our lives. No matter your age or gender, if you are a survivor of a traumatic experience, this book is here to help you in a way that won't burden you or bring you down. I will remind you what a unique and resilient person you are and how, if you embrace this healing journey, you can be the best possible version of yourself.

WE ARE NOT JUST OUR MINDS: HOW TRAUMA IMPACTS OUR BODY AND HEALTH

Trauma is an experience all humans have in common and something we all can relate to. Sometimes this can be obvious: We are in a car accident, or we lose a loved one unexpectedly—this can be a traumatic experience for us, but sometimes, the trauma is not so obvious. Maybe we have encountered conflict with a colleague at work; perhaps someone has insulted or belittled us. It may not sound like much, but these small things can also be traumatic experiences. The risk of trauma is something we live through every day. Our reaction to trauma varies from person to person because it is dependent on how each person's brain reacts to those situations—both at the time of the event and in the future.

The problem is that if trauma is not addressed, then it isn't just our brain that is impacted but our whole bodies. The effects of trauma can severely impact our well-being and health. It can affect everything from your digestion to your heart rate. It is important to remember that trauma is not something that only affects our mind: It can affect our whole body and any area of our health. Of course, it is essential that we clear the trauma from our bodies and learn to heal. Otherwise, it can lead to chronic illness. Trauma has led to illnesses such as type 2 diabetes, rheumatoid arthritis, and heart disease (Richmond, 2018). My dad was diagnosed with rheumatoid arthritis late in his life. Knowing what I know about trauma now, I wonder whether that was linked to his wife (my mother) dying. They had been together for a very long time. To say it was a shock to his system when she died would be an understatement. If only I had known about somatic healing therapy at the time, maybe I could have been more helpful to my dad in helping him navigate that traumatic experience. We all have different reactions, though, so I do want to reassure you that just because you have suffered a traumatic experience, it does not immediately mean you will suffer illness. But it does have the potential to do that if not addressed.

Something like trauma, often seen as a mental aspect, manifests itself in physical reactions such as headaches, muscle tension, fatigue, and stomach trouble (Richmond, 2018). It's the kind of constant physical pain that none of us want to endure unless we have to. It also plays out in our emotions and feelings. Some of us may feel bewildered; some may feel completely isolated; some feel trapped; some feel hopeless and as if they have no control over themselves; or some may stop feeling and stop caring about them-selves and others altogether. Trauma may start in the brain, but it can affect our whole being if we don't learn to heal from it. That's the information I am going to attempt to provide to you. By following the advice and exercises provided in this book, you can begin your healing journey and learn to transform your life so that the past no longer dominates it. It's time for you to stop remembering the past and concentrate on shaping your future instead.

IF YOU UNDERSTAND SOMATIC THERAPY, THEN YOU UNDERSTAND HOW TO ALTER YOUR EXISTENCE FOREVER

The word "somatic" originally comes from the Greek word *soma* which means "living body" (Erdelyi, 2019). This look at the word's origin gives you a good idea of what somatic therapy is. It is about listening to your body as well as your mind and making the connection between the two. By listening to the body and learning to heal the body, you will, in turn, heal your mind. The thinking behind somatic therapy is that much of what we suffer from now is due to past trauma. Much of this trauma is thought to have become trapped within our nervous systems. The symptoms and effects of trauma we display physically result from the instability of our nervous systems caused by those past experiences.

Some may dismiss this belief as hocus-pocus. Science is backing up this theory that the body and mind are connected. Morrisey once sang in The Smith's song "Still Ill": "Does the body rule the mind or does the mind rule the body? I don't know" (Morrisey & Marr, 1984). However, the more scientific and medical research executed in this area, the more we realize that the mind and the body are interconnected, and pain can work both ways. For example, a study carried out in 2005 concluded that chronic back pain often resulted in things like anxiety and extreme emotional responses (Von Korff et al., 2005). A study in 2020 focused on how social pain, i.e., isolating yourself or negative experiences of interaction, can result in physical pain (Zhang et al., 2020). Therefore, somatic healing is used as a therapy because it addresses both the mind and the body. It also addresses our emotions and feelings. It doesn't just assume physical pain can only be healed by physical therapy or that mental health can only be addressed via psychological therapy.

SOMATIC PSYCHOLOGY AND PSYCHOTHERAPY

Now it's time to introduce somatic psychology and psychotherapy. Somatic psychology encompasses therapeutic and holistic methods regarding the body, of which somatic psychotherapy is the largest branch.

Somatic psychotherapy also embraces the therapeutic and holistic approach of somatic psychology. It looks to address issues with the body, mind, and emotions within the process of healing. The belief is that a person's thoughts, outlook, principles, and emotions can impact their physical well-being, and physical things like posture, exercise, and diet can impact a person mentally. Anyone who saw Morgan Spurlock's 2004 documentary *Super Size Me* will know that Morgan had many wide-ranging physical issues caused by dining at a well-known fast-food chain and also suffered extreme mood swings. His mental health and not just his physical health, deteriorated due to the experiment.

Somatic psychotherapy is a method rooted in the connection between the body and the mind. Believers in somatic psychotherapy see the mind and body all as one, and any therapy should address both of these factors. They believe that the mind and the body can move toward healing when given the right approach, environment, social interactions, encouragement, and respect. If so, then the mind and the body can regulate themselves to cope with the stresses and strains of life. Otherwise, the trauma is stored in the body and can impact things like posture, facial expressions, and body language. Traditional therapies like talk therapy can help with trauma, but also adding a holistic approach such as somatic therapeutic techniques can work wonders. The same is true of body therapies: These may address physical issues and even some psychological issues, but they do not resolve deep-seated mental health problems.

Often, William Reich gets credited with forming the ideas behind somatic healing. However, he benefited from being a student of Sigmund Freud, who himself developed early thoughts about what we now think of as somatic healing. Pierre Janet is also an early contributor to these kinds of thoughts and ideas. However, Reich developed these views into much more of a progressive concept. He believed that human instincts were naturally good. From that belief, he formed a theory that incorporated the body. Reich's 1933 book *Character Analysis* suggested that the body was affected by buried emotions and even a person's personality. This could result in tension in the muscles, posture, and the way a person moves. He referred to this idea as "body armor." Therefore, he concluded that to release emotions trapped deep inside the body, some kind of physical force had to be applied to the body (Bell, 2017). Although some of Reich's later ideas were rejected by the psychology profession, he had laid the cornerstones for somatic therapy. It is widely accepted now that the mind and the body are much more aligned and not separate entities as previously believed. Many professionals dealing in mental health now support a more holistic approach when dealing with those affected by trauma.

Somatic psychotherapy works by paying attention to the body's signals—not only what our mind tells us. It may be tension in the muscles—usually around the head, neck, and shoulders—or it can manifest as digestion issues, hormonal problems, or sexual dysfunction. Somatic psychotherapists will help a person listen to their body and become aware of these signals. They will then assign the

3

therapeutic technique they believe will best help to alleviate the problems. It could be such exercises as breathing techniques or something very physical like dance movement. The person may also discuss their behavioral habits and to note, in the future, the impact those habits have on any new thoughts and feelings that may crop up during somatic therapy.

Essentially, somatic therapy can help people with awareness of their bodies and minds and in assisting them with opening up and thinking more about their emotions and physical issues. As we will see in some later chapters, somatic therapy is very much becoming the norm for assisting those who have suffered post-traumatic stress disorder (PTSD). Understanding somatic therapy and including it into your routine can help address any number of issues such as dealing with stress, anxiety, and depression, assisting with relationship and interaction issues, or helping boost self-confidence and belief in oneself.

KEY SOMATIC THERAPY CONCEPTS

I will be discussing the key concepts contained in each chapter in much more detail as we go along. However, in this first chapter, I wanted to provide you with a brief outline of these essential concepts so that you will already have a basic understanding when we delve deeper into these ideas later.

Grounding

Grounding is a technique used on the body that enables one to feel themselves in the present moment. It uses the person's ability to sense their physical body, using their senses and feeling their feet on the ground. In essence, grounding is about managing the nervous system and learning to feel calm.

Boundary Development

Boundary development is all about the person concentrating on the here and now, giving them the tools to respond positively to their changing requirements, and setting clear boundaries. It enables a person to react to changing situations confidently and to establish a guard against becoming overwhelmed.

Self-Regulation

I think some people feel I could do with self-regulation when it comes to cakes or alcohol! Yet this concept is more to do with self-regulating your body, not necessarily your diet or your drinking habits (though self-regulating both is never a bad idea). It is the idea that the person stays aware and feels part of their body during deep emotions or sensations. The person learns to self-regulate any major physical sensibilities and can self-regulate them or respond appropriately at times of severe emotional impact.

Movement and Process

As I have outlined, somatic therapy is all about listening to one's body. This means that a person's posture, sense of space, and body language, such as gestures, can give an accurate understanding of the types of life experiences that a person may have been through. Movement can be something for a person to engage with to help with the issues they have.

Sequencing

Sequencing is all about how the tension built up by traumatic experiences may move around the body. For example, the tension may begin in the stomach. It may then move up the chest, which may tighten, and then move further up to the throat where, again, tightening may occur—making it difficult to breathe. Maybe the tension results in crying freely and tears coming out of the eyes, therefore bringing some release to the person and allowing them to breathe easier.

Titration

Titration is the procedure of encountering minor amounts of anguish while healing the person overall. A person will very slowly delve back into their past traumatic experiences, and as they do, the somatic therapist will check the responses and sensations in the body. They won't just keep an eye on the physical aspect: They will continue to talk to the person, but they will be watching out for things like difficulty in breathing, clenched fists, gnashing or grinding of teeth, or a difference in the sound of the voice.

Resourcing

Resourcing relates to the resources you can give a person to feel they have safe choices to make and do not become overwhelmed and anxious. The person will learn to identify places, people, and things to make them feel safe and calm. They will use these whenever they are feeling distressed. They will find out how to feel at peace with the world and what their body is feeling.

ARE THERE LIMITATIONS TO SOMATIC PSYCHOTHERAPY?

Although somatic psychotherapy is becoming more common as a therapy option for dealing with trauma, some concerns and limitations have been raised by those who oppose it. One such concern is touch therapy, which can sometimes be used as part of somatic therapy. Touch therapy is something many therapy professionals believe has ethical implications. Although it is recognized that some touch therapy can have a healing effect in reducing pain or tension, it is also recognized that touching some victims of abuse could trigger their trauma. There is also the possibility that just as touching may cause trauma to reoccur, it may also make some people very uncomfortable, or some may even find it arousing. This may mean it distracts from the purpose of the therapy. The patient may end up transferring feelings and emotions that relate to someone or something else onto the therapist; the reverse is also possible—the therapist places feelings and emotions not directly relevant to the patient on them. Therefore, both the therapist and the patient need to agree that touching is an acceptable part of the therapy, and the patient is willing to investigate and develop an awareness of their body. Not all body psychotherapy courses have been accredited in some countries, as it is considered that they do not meet all the scientific criteria required. Therefore, when searching out these specific types of courses, you do need to be aware of that scenario (Bell, 2017).

DIFFERENT TYPES OF TRAUMA THERAPY

Finally, in this chapter, I will outline some of the programs and procedures you can follow and take part in when it comes to somatic therapy. I will be discussing these in much more detail in the various chapters throughout the book, but this is to give you a flavor as to what might appeal to you or ones you might be specifically interested in—though all can benefit.

Art Therapy

Art therapy can be a useful way to treat trauma. It allows a person to create what they want and at the pace they want. Plus, it includes both visual and physical elements. The art then becomes a release of that trauma while also enabling a person to become more aware of their body and the sensations involved when touching things and creating.

Emotional Freedom Technique (EFT) Tapping

EFT uses similar principles to acupuncture. It believes there are specific points on the body related to organs or other internal parts of the body. Using your fingers and tapping on these points sends messages to the brain. This, in turn, can relieve the tension and pressure that has built up due to the negative experiences and emotions a person may have experienced.

Eye Movement Desensitization and Reprocessing (EMDR) Therapy

EMDR therapy works by the person reliving their trauma slowly and intermittently while the therapist instructs you to move your eyes. The thinking around this is that it is easier to cope with recalling terrible past experiences when your attention is diverted elsewhere. Having your attention distracted like this produces much less of a physical and emotional response to the trauma.

Energy Psychology

EFT is a type of energy psychology. It involves using acupuncture-type methods to tap the body's energy points while the person undergoing the therapy focuses on traumatic events or experiences in their life.

Focusing Therapy

Focusing therapy is all about having that feeling in your body whenever you remember traumatic experiences—focusing on that feeling in the body so that it forms an image. That image can then be used to tell where the trauma is stuck and how to deal with it.

Gestalt Therapy

Gestalt therapy is very much about concentrating on the here and now. It intends to stop a person from constantly thinking only about the past. It encourages a person to be aware of the feelings and emotions they are currently having, and it advises how they can relate that to physical symptoms. There are various forms of Gestalt therapy which I will discuss in more detail later on.

Guided Imagery Therapy

"Imagine you're on a beach, and the waves are lapping at your feet." We have all heard this kind of thing when getting people to relax. That is what guided imagery therapy is: It uses images to help people free themselves from mental anguish and stress.

Mindfulness

Mindfulness is the practice of the awareness of thoughts and feelings as they appear without passing judgment on those thoughts.

Psychodrama

Psychodrama works on the basis that it enables the person to say or do whatever it is that is needed to let them heal from the trauma. This involves reliving the trauma, for which various techniques can be applied. I will discuss this in further detail later on in the book.

Sensorimotor Psychotherapy

This aspect of psychotherapy is centered around the body and how listening to it and understanding it can help heal our trauma.

Somatic Experiencing

Somatic experiencing is also about putting the body at the center—specifically the nervous system—and listening to what it is saying and responding accordingly.

Dance/Movement Therapy

As you can guess from its name, this form of therapy uses movement, often dance. The suggestion is that the person may be able to express themselves through dance and movement in a way they never could verbally; doing this can help heal mental health issues.

🦋 2 🦋

SOMATIC MINDFULNESS AND EXPERIENCING

SOMATIC MINDFULNESS

Somatic mindfulness is a vital part of somatic therapy. The awareness of your body and what it is doing in the here and now is a big fixture of somatic therapy—not how your body was feeling in the past or will be feeling in the future. Many of us do not listen to our bodies and are oblivious to what they are trying to tell us. You have the ability to remove yourself from what the nervous system is telling you. It may be telling you to feel anxious, defensive, or overwhelmed—whatever behavior you subconsciously feel most comfortable with—even if the reality is it makes you uncomfortable.

Mindfulness started as a Buddhist concept. It then slowly developed over the many centuries into something Western therapists and doctors often use to help with mental health.

There is an excellent example that Andrea Bell tells from her therapy experience. It involves a patient from a challenging background where he could not trust anyone. After a few sessions with him, for reasons that had nothing to do with the patient, she changed the furniture in her office to more, in her eyes, comfortable furniture. However, when he came in and sat down on the new, comfier, and more luxurious chair, he became immediately suspicious, questioning Andrea why she had changed the furniture and whether she was doing it on purpose to mess with his head. Once Andrea had explained the real reasons for changing it, the boy then relaxed and enjoyed the new chair's comfort. That shows you how we are often dictated to by our behaviors and experiences of the past that we forget to enjoy the present and then use it to suggest how the future might go. In this instance, the boy was under the assumption that the therapy sensations with Andrea were going to fail. Andrea then worked with the boy to distinguish what physical sensations he felt when he came into the room. He will then be able to note those reactions when he next gets them and learn to listen to them and think about whether that is the most appropriate response. The more he does that, the more his initial reaction to change should calm down and, slowly, no longer feel like a threat (Bell, 2018).

The other thing about mindfulness is that it teaches us how to stop judging ourselves. Instead of thinking about something we said or did wrong in the past while we are going about our daily lives, mindfulness teaches us not to judge ourselves so harshly. It assists us with trying not to worry about things in the past but concentrate and enjoy only the present.

We know this can work. If you have ever studied athletes before a race, you will see them going through various motions and rituals. All they are doing is practicing mindfulness to be well and truly in the present moment and, therefore, relaxed and calm—not having those doubtful, anxious thoughts run through their mind and show in their body through muscle tension. Those practicing mindfulness the most are usually the ones that win the race.

There is plenty of evidence that backs up the success of mindfulness in assisting with many issues. It can help cut down procrastination. One study showed that those competing in an intensive meditation course showed much improvement in that procrastination than those who did not undergo the course (Chambers et al., 2008). There are also several studies proclaiming the reduction of stress and anxiety as a result of practicing mindfulness. A 2010 study concluded that mindfulness effectively treated stress, anxiety, and other possible mood issues (Hoffman et al., 2010).

It does not stop there either. A 2009 study suggested that mindfulness could vastly improve your attention and focus. Those that took part in specific tests performed much better if they had been practicing mindfulness than those that had not (Moore & Malinowski, 2009).

Furthermore, a study from 2007 showed that those that had practiced mindfulness coped with seeing upsetting or emotionally inducing pictures far better than those that did not practice mindfulness. The study concluded that mindfulness could reduce the impact of things that tend to provoke an emotional response (Ortner et al., 2007).

It seems mindfulness not only has a good impact on yourself but also on your relationships with others. A 2007 study found that those who engaged in mindfulness were far better able to deal with the kind of conflict that crops up in romantic relationships; were more likely to be in a happy and satisfying relationship; and those that practiced mindfulness were able to communicate better than those that did not practice it (Barnes et al., 2007).

One of the by-products of the current pandemic and the many lockdowns occurring around the world is that it has resulted in much stress and anxiety. It has become almost impossible to enjoy the present because we constantly worry about what is just around the corner. However, somatic mindfulness is something you can introduce with ease to your daily routine; therefore, you can reduce the stress and anguish you may be feeling. It is not something that will take up your whole day. All you need are 20 to 30 minutes somewhere in your day to relax and take stock of yourself and the world around you. You can be doing other things while you begin your mindfulness practice. You can be brushing your teeth and thinking about your feet being firmly on the floor, the feeling of the toothbrush in your hand and on your teeth, and the movement of your arm up and down or side to side as you brush.

Many people have dishwashers these days, but I'm not one of them. A good side effect is that I can practice mindfulness while washing the dishes. I can concentrate on the feeling of the soapy water on my hands and the sounds of the cutlery against the dishes. Washing dishes is a great way to become aware of the sights and sounds and increase your awareness. If you are putting your clean clothes away, then take a moment to smell and feel them. You can even take some deep breaths and be aware of your breathing while you fold and put them away. If you are a gym rat (or just an occasional gym-goer), try running on the treadmill instead of looking at the TV on your next visit. Instead of listening to a thumping beat on your headphones, try to focus on the feeling of your feet on the treadmill as you move. Hone in on your breathing and how it quickens as your pace on the treadmill accelerates.

With that in mind, how do you practice mindfulness meditation specifically? Well, the first thing is to get yourself comfortable. Find the most comfortable seat in your house or sit on the floor if you prefer. Don't laugh: I know some people who prefer sitting on the floor rather than on a chair. Wherever you sit, you need to keep your back straight but not so you are stiff. You want to be able to stay relaxed. Your chosen place should be as quiet as possible as you don't want there to be any noise to distract you. You should wear as comfortable of clothing as you can—not too loose and not too tight, as you don't want anything that will distract you from your meditation. To begin with, maybe you want to see if you can fully meditate for five minutes, then try for 10 minutes, then 15 or 20 minutes, and finally 30 minutes.

To begin with, concentrate on your breath. Be aware of your breathing. Notice the feeling of your diaphragm moving in and out. Notice the air coming in and out of your nostrils and mouth. You may even detect the drop in temperature when you let your breaths out compared to when you are breathing in.

The point of mindful meditation is not necessarily to completely stop your thoughts but to be aware of them and take notice as they occur. You don't need to try to ignore them or suppress them, but note them and keep calm, using your breathing to stop your mind from running away with you. You should note each thought and let it go—like factory products on a conveyor belt. You can do this as many times as you need to throughout your meditation.

If you do find your mind going off in different directions and you start to feel anxious or panicky, then take note of your thoughts and what caused you the stress. Then return to your breathing— deep, slow breaths. Don't judge yourself if this happens often. There are so many gizmos and gimmicks to distract us in the modern world. We are just not used to being quiet and in the present and aware, so don't be harsh on yourself. Mindfulness is all about getting back to your breathing and concentrating on living in the moment.

As you can see, you can easily practice this mindfulness at home. You don't need to be in a therapist's office to carry it out. If you are struggling, then there are thousands of videos on YouTube and many apps you can download to help you with your practice.

SOMATIC EXPERIENCING

Peter Levine specifically developed somatic experiencing (SE) to address those suffering from trauma. Levine was inspired after seeing animals that are often preyed upon quickly recover from any potential attack. They went through a physical process to release the nervous energy built up during the threat. Levine suggested that humans don't have that physical release; the trauma remains in their minds and leads to thoughts of anxiety, embarrassment, and many other hazardous feelings. The release that Levine believes nature requires does not occur sporadically in humans. Somatic experiencing is the answer to that—it helps humans process the trauma they have suffered that has become trapped inside them (Osadchey, 2018).

A human's nervous system leaps into action whenever we find ourselves in a dangerous situation, deciding our fight-flight-freeze response. It does this almost instinctively without us needing to think. However, the trouble is that when someone goes through a traumatic experience, particularly if that experience is buried and not released, the nervous system can start to go rogue. It starts to behave as though the person is constantly under threat of attack—every situation becomes a potentially traumatic one. Somatic experiencing believes that burying the trauma results in the kind of symptoms we often see, such as anxiety, shame, and embarrassment. If the body is allowed the opportunity to truly process the traumatic experience it has been through, then these symptoms do not come out to play in the long term. Somatic experiencing is very much about getting the body and nervous system to, once again, self-regulate themselves and find harmony and balance in the body.

Somatic experiencing concentrates on the feelings and sensations that occur in the body—becoming aware of them and understanding them. This can be quite intimidating for many people, as they have never thought about their body in this way; however, it can be very rewarding. Once you have become used to these feelings and sensations, you can start to note them, and when they occur in the future, you can prevent your mind from suppressing them. This is where the harmony between your brain and your body comes into play to allow the physical release of the trauma you need to allow yourself to heal.

As with all somatic healing therapy, research and evidence in this area is still new, so there is no conclusive proof. Still, scientific evidence that SE positively impacts those who have suffered trauma is growing. Although a study from 2017 used only a small sample of people, it found that SE is an effective treatment—specifically for those with PTSD (Brom et al, 2017).

Here are some straightforward and easy-to-do somatic experiencing exercises for you to do at home. You should begin to see if this form of therapy suits you and makes a positive difference. It would be best if you tried to manage at least one minute with exercise—ideally, considerably longer than that.

- **1:** Sit in your favorite comfy chair and take notice of how everything feels. Think about how your feet are planted on the floor; move them to and fro until you feel the floor is just an extension of your feet. Then, think about how your back and bottom feel on the chair or how the chair supports you. If you are leaning forward in the chair, then make sure you lean back and allow the chair to support you. Wriggle around in your chair until you reach your optimum comfort zone. Take some time to appreciate the comfort of the chair, the way it supports you, and the way the floor supports your feet. Take a peek around the room and outside your window, if you need to, and look for something that calms you and makes you feel happy—it could be a painting you have hanging on a wall or the walls themselves. It could be the trees and bushes outside; maybe the birds are chirping and playing in them. Perhaps it's the carpet on the floor. Whatever it may be, take the time to appreciate and enjoy them and the feelings they bring. Now that you've done all this, how do you feel about your comfort, both physically and emotionally? If you take your time with this exercise, it really can make a difference in calming down your nervous system and bringing some harmony to your body and emotions.
- **2:** For the second exercise, take a moment to take everything in—all of your surroundings and how you are

feeling. Then, take your right hand and put it just below your left armpit, clutching the side of your chest. Now, take your left hand and put it on your right bicep, elbow, or shoulder—whatever is easiest. At this juncture, take some time to think about how this makes you feel. Is your body cold or warm under your hands? Are your clothes soft, or are they more of a rough fabric? Is there anything else you are noticing? Maybe you can feel your heart beating; perhaps you are aware of your breathing. Do you find doing this satisfying? Does it bring some comfort wrapping your hands on your body like this? Then, see how the rest of your body responds to this kind of physical touch. Try the same thing with your legs. Now, compare what you notice about your surroundings and how your body feels with what you noted at the beginning of the exercise. In times of anxiety or stress, this type of exercise can bring back some comfort and peace to your body through your physical touch.

- **3:** One of the best exercises is to remember a time when someone showed you kindness. Even in the toughest of worlds and lives, there is at least one person who, at some point, shows us kindness. If we are lucky, there are many people throughout our lives. Try to remember those times when someone demonstrated their kindness to you. Remember the words they said, their hand gestures, their facial expressions, and everything that was part of that kindness act. As you remember this moment, take note of how your body responds to this memory—everything you are seeing, hearing, and feeling. It's almost like you have transported yourself back in time to that very moment. Now, compare what you felt at the time with what you are feeling now as you remember the experience. If any negative memories come through as a result of this remembrance, then try to place them in an imaginary folder and concentrate only on the memory of the act of kindness. At the end of the exercise, note how you are feeling now, how your body is feeling, and how you feel about your surroundings. This is an excellent way of calming yourself and remembering that not everyone is out to get you. You do not need to feel stressed about everyone you come into contact with; there are kind people out there ready to be kind to you.

- **4:** As with the start of most of these exercises, first, take note of your surroundings and your general feelings and emotions. Then, try to remember within the last 24 hours (or longer if you need to) when you last truly felt like yourself or the person you want to be. Recall this moment in as much detail as possible—almost as if you were living through it again. Take note of what you felt during that moment and what was occurring with your five senses. Then, again, remember when you were last most like yourself or the person you aim to be but this time, within the last few weeks. Again, try to recall as much detail as possible as though you were going through it again, and note how your body felt during that moment. Then, as usual, at the end of the exercise, see how you feel about your surroundings, general feelings, and emotions compared to how you felt at the start. This exercise is good at bringing you back to yourself, away from all the confusion and madness that you sometimes feel in the world.

- **5:** This exercise involves making some vocal noises, so it may be wise to go somewhere where you are truly alone before you carry out this exercise. As always, start by taking notice of your surroundings and your general emotions and feelings. Then, consider the kind of sound that a foghorn makes. Take a very deep breath, and attempt to make the sound of a foghorn. The sound needs to be a low-enough pitch so that you feel it reverberate around your body. See how far you can feel it down into your body—perhaps even down to the very bottom of your belly and possibly to your thighs. As you feel the sound end (it is often described as the "voo" sound), then let your next breath occur naturally. You can take your time; there is no need to rush the breath. If you feel comforted and in harmony, then stay with that feeling. For some people, though, making the foghorn sound can have an unsettling effect, so if that is the case with you, go back to one of the other exercises to regain your sense of harmony. If you found the foghorn sound comforting, then try it again. Do you feel even more comforted and in harmony? I would not suggest doing the sound more than three times, though. As with the end of the other exercises, how do you feel now? Compare it with how you felt at the start of the exercise. This can be an excellent exercise to help settle the body's core. As the sound reverberates around your body, this can help the muscles relax and release any tension you may be feeling.

THE HEALING POWER OF BREATH—SOMATIC BREATHWORK

We all take breathing for granted. It just so happens that we don't have to think about it at all, but that is part of the problem. We are not breathing as deeply as we should; our diaphragms are getting uptight and arent relaxed. By concentrating on breathing, we take care of ourselves both physically and mentally. We can control our breathing; we will breathe at the rate we choose. When we breathe, we also get the opportunity to be aware of our bodies and how they are feeling.

It is believed that breathing significantly impacts your blood pressure, your heart rate, and the arteries' ability to let blood flow through them. No wonder our breathing is one of the first things to get out of control when we are anxious or stressed. It's also believed that breathing deeply can lead to one being in a much better mood. People have also reported having a better night's sleep with fewer occurrences of waking up in the night. It does depend, though; just doing a minute here or there will have much less impact than conducting 30 minutes of breathing deeply day after day. Results for lowering blood pressure were still successful a month later for those that could stay regimented. It is perhaps common sense, but breathing in more oxygen gets the oxygen flowing through your blood cells and nerve tissues. For those that participated in deep breathing, it was reported that oxygen utilization increased by 37% (Hadley, 2017). A 2017 study also found that blood pressure was lowered using deep breathing for those with hypertension (Janet & Gowri, 2017). A 2019 study backed the theory that slow, deep breathing was a better tool for fighting insomnia than hypnosis or some pharmaceutical options (Jerath et al., 2019).

As with all somatic therapy, somatic breathing is all about taking notice of our body and how it works. It's about paying attention to the feeling of your stomach and belly contracting in and out and your rib area and chest as you breathe. Through somatic breathing, you also become so much more aware of your jaw, throat, diaphragm, and shoulders in the movement and motion of breathing. If we concentrate on our breathing and what our body is doing, we stop our minds racing away with all their concerns and worries. We start to truly live in the present moment and stop to smell the roses—or breathe in the aroma.

You can conduct somatic breathing, either sitting up or lying down on your back. You are aware of the breaths you take. This isn't the same as usual involuntary breathing, which happens without you even thinking about it. There is no break between breathing in and breathing out, and the breath can occur through the nose or the mouth. This kind of breathing should allow you to release some of the physical tension within. When you learn to breathe using your diaphragm and to relax when you breathe out, then this has the potential to release much deeper feelings and emotions. I will discuss diaphragm breathing later on in this chapter.

Although somatic breathing can be helpful to those suffering from PTSD, breathing can be one of the things that trigger PTSD symptoms. If you have PTSD and are thinking of investigating breathwork, you need to take extra care and remember that it is at your own risk, and you are responsible for your own health and well-being. If you ever have any doubt, you should seek a medical professional's help.

Here's a straightforward breathing exercise for you to follow:

- Take a normal breath. You should become aware that you want to take a deeper breath, equivalent to when you sigh.
- Breathe out. This should be for six to eight seconds, and you almost completely exhale.
- Gently hold still so that you are holding your breath out.
- At this point, concentrate on what it feels like to need to take another breath. What that sensation is physically, and where you are feeling it in your body. Linger on these sensations and feelings for a moment.
- The more interest you have in these feelings and sensations, the more you will find you can hold your breath.
- Once the need to breathe in again becomes obvious, note the feeling of it, and note that you can give in to it or keep holding your breath out for a few more seconds. Then breathe back in when you want to. Thus, you are now controlling your breathing—not your subconscious.
- Repeat this exercise for five minutes.

You may well have heard of the diaphragm, but you probably don't ever pay attention to it or know precisely what or where it is. Well, the diaphragm is a major muscle that exists just below your lung area, and it assists with ensuring air moves in and out of the lungs. In fact, the diaphragm is used in 80% of breathing. Breathing is much more efficient when the diaphragm is being used than when additional muscles are used (Diaphragmatic Breathing Exercises, n.d.). When a person breathes in, the diaphragm shrinks and heads downward, whereas when a person breathes out, the diaphragm loosens and heads upward, assisting in pushing the air out of the lungs. Considering that the average human will breathe 23,000 breaths a day, which works out to eight million a year, we can see just how important a muscle the diaphragm is (Diaphragmatic Breathing: Everything, n.d.).

When we breathe without thinking, this rarely uses the full capability of the lungs and is known as shallow breathing. However, diaphragmatic breathing uses deep breathing to make full use of this capability. It can also sometimes be known as "belly breathing." This is because it makes full use of the stomach and the abdominal muscles as well as the diaphragm with each breath. This involves consciously moving the diaphragm down when you breathe in, ensuring that the lungs fill with air much more efficiently. A person should realize that their stomach is moving up and down; they should feel their stomach being pulled tighter and relaxing rather than just feeling it in their chest and shoulders as you would with shallow breathing.

If you want to check whether you tend to breathe with your diaphragm or your chest, place your right hand on your chest and your left hand on your stomach and breathe. If your right-hand rises first, you are using your chest to breathe. If your left-hand rises first, you are using your diaphragm. I have noticed that when I am hunched over my desk at home on the laptop and stop to do that test, it is my right hand that rises first. If I sit up straight in my chair, the left-hand rises first. The amount of time people spend sitting in positions with bad posture is a concern of doctors and scientists. It leads to symptoms such as a bad back and causes one to use shallow breathing. This prevents one from getting enough oxygen into the body. No wonder I tend to go a bit light-headed after a while when I'm crouched over my computer.

You only need to practice diaphragmatic breathing for up to 10 minutes, and ideally, this should be for three to four times throughout the day. You should be able to find a moment while at home to lie down and practice your breathing. You want to try and find somewhere free from distractions, so stay away from the TV and leave your smartphone in a different room. Leave your partner/children/pets in a separate room. You want to ensure you will remain free from interruption while you carry out your breathing exercises. As with all somatic techniques, you want to concentrate on what your body is feeling as you experience your breathing.

If you find it useful, you can set an alarm to know when to take a break and carry out your exercises. It is often useful to remember you are always breathing, so this is not exactly going out of your way to do something; you are already doing it—you just need to concentrate and notice it.

There are many different versions of diaphragmatic breathing, but to carry out the most basic version, you need to do the following:

- Find a flat surface on which to lie down. I think for most people, that is likely to be the floor. Place a pillow or cushion under your head and also underneath your knees. The pillows and cushions are not essential, but if you have them, they are good to use as they will help keep your body in as comfortable a position as possible.
- Put one hand toward the top of your chest in the middle area.
- Put your other hand on your stomach, just below the ribcage but above the diaphragm.
- Breathe in through your nostrils only, pulling the air down toward your stomach. The stomach should move up toward the resistance of your hand, while your chest movement should be limited.
- Breathe out through your mouth, but don't open your mouth fully. Keep your lips tight together still. Your stomach should relax and go back in, and, again, there should not be any movement in your chest.

As with anything new, diaphragmatic breathing can feel odd at first, or it may feel like hard work. However, as with anything in life, the more you practice, the easier it should get. You may want to count a number in your head with each breath. Sometimes, this can help a person relax further and can help with knowing how many breaths you have completed. It may also help with keeping you from getting too easily distracted.

When you feel you have mastered this lying down, you can advance to practicing it sitting down or even standing up. This increases your opportunity as to when and where you can practice it. It means you can even do it when sitting at your desk at work, standing in a line, watching TV, sitting on a bus, or anything you can imagine. Once you can successfully practice sitting up and standing up, it opens a whole new world of opportunity and chance for you to carry out your practice. Be careful that when you do advance to that, you must ensure that your head, neck, and shoulders move as little as possible when sitting or standing. Don't be hard on yourself if things aren't going quite as you hoped or the breathing doesn't seem to be working. This is practice. The more you do it and get used to it, the better you will become and feel comfortable. No one else is judging you on how you do, so don't judge yourself. You'll get there with plenty of practice. You have to continue to do it regularly as well. Your body has the memory of a goldfish rather than an elephant when it comes to diaphragmatic breathing, so it won't remember when you did it in the past. You need to keep regularly practicing for it to take effect.

Why would you want to practice diaphragmatic breathing? Well, for a start, the diaphragm is a muscle, so you are strengthening that muscle just by doing this exercise. That alone makes it worthwhile, but other benefits cited include strengthening your core and lowering your heart rate and blood pressure (Johnson, 2020).

The great thing about diaphragmatic breathing is that evidence is mounting to suggest it can positively help alleviate stress and anxiety. A 2017 study noted that it reduced stress hormones in the body, therefore potentially also reducing the feelings of stress and anxiety in a person (Ma et al., 2017). This was further solidified by a 2019 review of studies and evidence that concluded that diaphragmatic breathing can be used as a tool for stress reduction (Hopper et al., 2019).

However, suppose someone with anxiety tries diaphragmatic breathing and finds it does not work. In that case, it may make them more anxious, so always seek out the assistance of a medical professional before embarking on these types of exercises.

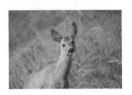

4

EMPOWER YOURSELF BY UNDERSTANDING PTSD AND ATTACHMENT TRAUMA

P ost-traumatic stress disorder (PTSD) can occur in individuals after living through or being party to a traumatic event. PTSD usually occurs when people have been involved in truly terrible events and not just minor traumatic occurrences. It is also fair to say that just because someone suffers trauma doesn't mean they will develop PTSD: It depends on each individual. Symptoms of PTSD can include flashbacks, an inability to think about anything other than the event, and anxiety on a very serious level. Sometimes, these symptoms can occur within a month of an event; sometimes, they occur several years after the event.

Complex post-traumatic stress disorder (CPTSD) is best explained as a sufferer of PTSD displaying additional symptoms following a traumatic event. You may find it hard to keep your emotions in check; you may feel very angry at the world; you may find it difficult to trust anyone or anything; you may feel like something is missing, or you feel you are not worth anything, and that nobody else in the world could possibly understand you or the way you are feeling. All this can lead to disassociating yourself from relationships or friendships, and it can take on physical pain, including headaches and chest pain. Complex PTSD includes flashbacks like

PTSD, but they are more emotional flashbacks so that you don't just re-experience the event itself but all of the emotions you felt at the time. You then display those feelings in the present, even though the flashback is causing those emotions.

Attachment trauma that occurs early in a child's life, usually from neglect and abuse, can stem from something like separation from a caregiver due to medical concerns or death. It is not always the case that attachment trauma immediately directs back to the parents, and the trauma is the parents' fault. Trauma can come from many different directions and people, so we should take that into consideration. Since we cannot recall memories before the age of four or five, we think we cannot remember the traumatic events. However, our brain and body have remembered it even if our memory cannot. These feelings and emotions can then occur later in life. The trauma will usually show up in things like a fear of relationships, a constant sense of shame, or that the person is unworthy of somebody else's love. As the person may have no memory of why this occurred, it can make it much more challenging to treat than some of the other traumas.

As I alluded to earlier, not everyone will develop PTSD, CPTSD, or attachment trauma from traumatic events. Some will suffer minor trauma, and some will not suffer anything at all, though it is estimated that 70% of adults in America have suffered a traumatic event at some point in their lives (Eckelkamp, 2019). Trauma isn't just something that happens to other people; we are all likely to face it in our lives. Even general trauma requires addressing; otherwise, it can result in mental and physical issues. Trauma can be defined as anything that results in us being stuck in a physical, emotional, or behavioral pattern (Cutler, n.d.). Processing and getting over the trauma often ends up being interrupted; hence the trauma ends up stored in our bodies, and we never truly release it. Stored trauma can often lead to physical pain and the psychological anguish that comes along with it.

That is where somatic healing and therapy come in. Things like deep breathing, somatic experiencing, and movement can help relieve that stuck trauma in your body as you gently and slowly begin to release the tension. Perhaps these methods will allow your brain to process things you had long consigned to your brain's "Recycle Bin."

It's a sad cycle that disability and chronic illness can cause short-term and long-term trauma, but then those who suffer trauma, if not treated correctly, end up developing physical conditions and symptoms. Therefore, someone who develops chronic illness can also be traumatized by it, which in turn, if they are not able to release that trauma, may end up making them feel even more ill and develop further physical pain.

When individuals are diagnosed with a disability or a chronic illness, this can be a very traumatic event. All sorts of over-whelming feelings are likely to be going through a person, and because people start talking about treatment or next steps, the person doesn't always get the chance to process that trauma. It's a worrying estimation that between 12% and 25% of those who develop life-threatening illnesses go on to develop PTSD (Virant, 2019). It is no surprise that people who go through these types of experiences often develop a fear of hospitals or doctors. Most worryingly, it can develop into a complete mistrust of doctors and a wish to avoid having anything to do with the illness. For example, the afflicted individual starts "forgetting" to take their medication or turn up for appointments. Disability and chronic illness will often make a person question their place in the world and what they had always believed to be true. It makes them think about death, how vulnerable we all are, and how helpless we believe we may be. Having to go through emotions and experiences like this, it is not surprising that those with illnesses and disabilities develop trauma.

As mentioned when I began discussing CPTSD, relationships are all too often one of the things severely impacted by those suffering from trauma. It is understandable that a person suffering from trauma may find it hard to form long-lasting relationships. They may well feel danger is around every corner, and trusting either new friends or old friends can become exceptionally difficult. The anger that a person may feel due to losing control over the life they believe they may have lost or the helplessness they feel can link back to chronic illness. This can involve the individual lashing out at those close to them. The person feels under threat from everyone, therefore lashing out and becoming a defense mechanism. They can't hurt you if you hurt them first.

Depending on the type of trauma one is going through and their traumatic experience, one might go through feelings of shame, feeling as if they are not worthy of another's love, or feeling entirely unlovable. They may even feel guilty about what happened, that somehow the event was their fault, or they deserved it rather than realizing the blame lies with the perpetrator. Having gone through such traumatic events, the person believes nobody else can understand them, so they go through the burden alone and do not share with the people closest to them. Although the following are fictional accounts, I am about to use them as examples. I have no doubt the writers researched thoroughly about trauma survivors in order to make sure their characters behaved authentically. The first example is a plot line from a popular modern drama show. In one example, the character, June, has finally escaped into Canada from Gilead, where all her traumatic experiences occurred. She seems fairly incapable of sharing her experiences with anyone. Still, the person she definitely seems incapable of sharing her events with is her husband, who has been in Canada while she was in Gilead (Miller et al., 2017–present). Another example is from a famous Australian soap opera, where one of the characters, Marilyn, goes through a shared traumatic event with other characters but not her husband. Following this event, she feels the only person she can talk to about it is one of the other characters who went through the same thing. She becomes ever more distant from her husband, who she feels cannot understand what she went through or what she is feeling, eventually culminating in a divorce—although that is not the only reason they divorce (Holmes & McGauran, 1988–present). These two fictional examples are good at highlighting exactly the kinds of feelings and emotions a person who has been through trauma might exhibit. They suggest how trauma may impact their relationships with those closest to them.

Further than that, it may make the person who has encountered trauma ultimately isolate themselves. Sadly, in the current pandemic climate, that is something we are all doing. However, those that have suffered trauma will do it on purpose—putting distance between their partners, friends, families, and colleagues and maybe even become distant from life itself. They're going through detachment and may have no feelings about anything—almost becoming numb to anything around them. Some sufferers may become highly anxious and start showing trauma symptoms any time there is any possibility of them becoming rejected—say, by a potential partner. Others may go the other way and become entirely dependent on someone or become overprotective of their loved ones. If this includes children, then it may start to impact the child's life, as the child is not allowed to do anything that may put them in even the slightest harm. This pertains to just about anything and everything. Getting out of bed in the morning is a risk. There is nothing in life where there is no risk, so this can become problematic if a parent's trauma manifests itself in this way. Some people may find it extremely difficult to have any kind of physical relationship, to be able to place themselves in intimate situations, or find sexual relationships satisfactory. All of the feelings, emotions, and behaviors I have outlined can be bewildering and upsetting, but they are all normal things to think and feel if you have been through trauma. You should not castigate yourself any further. Understandably, trauma can result in these kinds of issues; you should not feel any worse about yourself because you can't make your relationship work after having been through trauma.

THE FIGHT, FLIGHT, FREEZE, OR FAWN RESPONSE

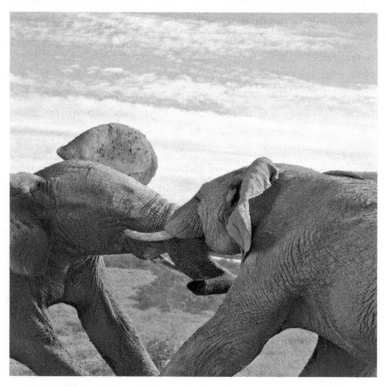

The fight, flight, freeze, or fawn responses are our responses when we encounter what we think is a threat or a danger to us. We do it automatically and subconsciously without even thinking about it. Flight, flight, and freeze are well-known responses, but fawn is also a possible response.

Flight is our wish to run away or flee from the situation that is causing us danger. This is a perfectly acceptable reaction and is not in any way cowardly as some posturing courageous people may view it as. After all, if you're stuck in a burning building, the best response is to get the heck out. Signs that you might be in flight mode include the following:

- Your legs feel very fidgety or restless.
- Your fingers, toes, ears, and nose (or any combination of those) become numb.
- Your eyes move around a lot or become dilated.
- Your muscles and body tense up.
- You feel like a prisoner and feel trapped.

Fight is exactly what it suggests: It becomes an aggressive response to the situation. Some indicators you may be in a "fight" mode include the following:

- You burst into tears.
- You have an overwhelming desire to punch something or somebody.
- You are grinding your teeth, or you feel your jaw tightening.
- You feel like stomping your feet or kicking something or somebody.
- You feel a deep, burning sense of anger.
- You imagine the possibility of harming someone— possibly even yourself.
- You feel pain or a burning sensation in the pit of your stomach.

Fight mode means you typically attack the source of the danger. This can be a very beneficial reaction unless the source you are attacking is capable of causing much more damage to you than you are to them.

The freeze response is best explained as becoming incapable of doing anything in the face of danger and literally freezing. It's like the phrase when a "deer is caught in the headlights." When a deer is in the middle of the highway and sees a car coming toward it, it freezes, and the car either swerves to avoid it or, sadly, hits it. Maybe you've even done this yourself: I know I have. I've stepped out on the road without paying attention, and when I see the car coming toward me rather than running out of the road, I just freeze, and I only survive because the driver stops the car in time. Some indicators you have gone into a freeze response include the following:

- Your body feels cold.
- Your body feels numb.
- You go very white—particularly in the face.
- Your legs feel like lead, and it is difficult to move your body.
- You feel very nervous and anxious.
- Your heart rate decreases, and you can feel it beating.

But what about the fawn response? This is a much lesser-known response. This response is where we will undertake anything or do anything to appease the situation. This can be particularly prevalent among those who have suffered childhood trauma. There was likely someone in their life that they would do or say anything to just to avoid whatever traumatic scenario would play out if they didn't. This type of fawn response is then often carried through to adulthood, and the person could end up in some unhealthy relationships and situations as a result.

Due to the fawn response often first occurring in childhood, it can make it difficult for a person to recognize what is happening when they are an adult. Hence, it is their default response to dangerous situations. However, there are some giveaway signals that you (or someone) could demonstrate with the fawn response:

- To see how you feel in a relationship or situation, you will view how other people feel.
- Even when alone, you find it tricky to work out what you are feeling.

- You feel like you do not have an individual personality, character, or identity.
- You are always trying to please everybody else in your life rather than concentrating and putting yourself first.
- Whenever conflict arises, your first action is to try and please or give in to the angry or annoyed person.
- You disregard your own beliefs or views and instead accept only the views of those around you as being true.
- You may find you provide strange emotional responses to things that, on the surface, don't appear to matter. For example, you could have an angry response to a stranger, or you could suddenly find yourself with a feeling of sadness, which can occur throughout the day.
- You feel guilty and angry at yourself much of the time.
- You find it difficult to say "no" to anyone.
- Everything can become too much for you, yet you will still take on more if requested.
- It is not easy to define boundaries, and you find that you are often being taken advantage of in a relationship.
- You are not happy, unsure, or even scared when asked to give your own opinion.

For those suffering from PTSD, CPTSD, or attachment trauma, there is already a level of self-blame and recrimination that can only worsen if the default response to danger is a fawn response. That is one of the many reasons it is essential to learn why these responses occur and what we can do to switch them off.

There is also talk of a fifth response known as "flop." This is where a person becomes utterly unresponsive to the occurring situation and may even lose consciousness. The term comes from the way the body flops like a rag doll.

All of these responses are perfectly natural, and people will demonstrate different reactions at different times. However, it can become concerning when we perceive threats where there are none, or we make the wrong response to the situation. These types of problems usually occur when we have become stuck in these responses because of past trauma that we have undergone. To get ourselves free from these trapped responses, we need to become more aware of how to feel safe, comforted, and without tension within our bodies. We should use exercises that allow us to safely release some of that trauma, which should mean less dependence on our fight, flight, freeze, or fawn responses.

Peter Levine based his "Somatic Experiencing" theory and work around the fact that he had observed animals in the wild. Despite being constantly in danger from predators, being chased by predators, and sometimes being momentarily captured but escaping, the animals did not suffer trauma. They carried on their life like they always had. Levine noted that animals after such an episode tended to shake and tremble, so he formed the belief that wild animals were able to "shake off" their trauma, whereas humans had lost this ability. As humans have lost the ability to shake off the trauma, trauma can end up stuck in the body, and only with the help of somatic therapy can it slowly and carefully be released (Osadchey, 2018).

I will provide you with a very simple exercise to follow so that you can switch off those fight-or-flight responses and remain calm and rational. It's a simple grounding exercise, and like all somatic healing exercises, it works from the body up to the brain rather than the other way around. This makes sense because we cannot think ourselves out of these situations or out of feeling anxious, but we can get our body to relax, be calm, and tell our brain that all is well.

GROUNDING EXERCISE

As going into fight-or-flight mode can make you feel almost detached from your body or as though your body is incapable of doing what you want it to, one way to get you back to a less anxious state is to reunite your brain with your body. One way to do this is by putting something hot or cold against your body. Obviously, be careful not to scold yourself or give yourself frostbite. If you put something mildly hot or cold on your body, it should reunite you with your body as you let your brain concentrate on what the sensations you're feeling are rather than focusing on false or impending dangers.

ATTACHMENT TRAUMA

I briefly mentioned attachment trauma at the beginning of this chapter, and I'm now going to cover it in much more detail in this section.

Attachment trauma occurs when there is an interruption to the normal bonding processes between a baby or a child and their principal caregivers—whether that be a parent or other guardian. That can be the result of abuse or neglect, but it can just be a general lack of affection or abandonment that was not the caregiver's fault.

Psychology identifies four main styles of attachment that a child may experience early in life with their caregiver. Depending on these styles, they will likely affect the child when they have grown into an adult:

- **1: Security:** People who feel secure grew up with attentive, loving, and sensitive caregivers sensitive to their child's needs. If a person obtains the security attachment, then they are likely to feel comfortable showing and speaking their emotions, will display confidence in themselves in relationships and will be able to face difficult situations and unhappy feelings in a healthy manner.
- **2: Avoidance:** Avoidant attachment occurs when a caregiver does not respond or is not sensitive to a child when hurt or in anguish. Children who experience this

type of attachment are likely to grow up not showing their emotions and will not look to their caregiver to provide assurance and comfort. As adults, they are likely to be distant in relationships and not capable of showing or speaking about their emotions.

- **3: Resistance:** A resistant attachment will develop if the caregiver is not consistent or not predictable in the way they respond to a child's anguish or upset. The child may use extreme methods to get the appropriate response from the caregiver. In adulthood, this can display itself as someone who is very needy and clingy in a relationship and is not secure at all in believing their partner loves them.

- **4: Disorganization:** A disorganized attachment will form when a caregiver's behavior is unusual or, in some way, scary. The child does not know what to do to get the comfort and assurance they require. In adulthood, this can lead to relationships full of conflict and arguments.

- The first style of attachment, security, will allow children to develop healthily and become more likely to have healthy relationships in later years. The other styles will result in an incomplete attachment being formed and will likely cause unhealthy relationships and other issues in adulthood.

When the unhealthy styles occur, this can result in traumatic events for a child. Of course, this can include severe events like abuse and extreme neglect, but it can also be something as simple as a child hurting themselves and crying as the caregiver ignores them (whether this is on purpose or not). This can result in a traumatic event for the child. One rare incident in a child's life may not result in attachment trauma, but if this is a consistent pattern, then that can cause long-lasting trauma into adulthood.

However, it doesn't have to be anything the caregiver has done that may cause the failure of the attachment to occur. The caregiver might have unfortunately died, the bond broken, and the secure attachment cannot be developed. It is not always as simple as being the caregiver's fault when attachment trauma occurs.

A person suffering from attachment trauma may find that they are more likely to suffer from stress and anxiety, find it difficult to emote, have trouble sleeping, isolate themselves, or have mental health issues.

If you do suffer from attachment trauma, I will give you an exercise to follow, but please be careful. This exercise can bring up some powerful emotions and feelings. If you think that will be too much for you at this stage, then that is perfectly understandable; you should leave this exercise alone until you are ready or visit a professional therapist.

ATTACHMENT TRAUMA EXERCISE

First of all, find yourself a hard floor if you can. You can do this exercise on carpet, but it makes it trickier. Once you have found the relevant floor, take your socks off. You should then lie flat on the floor so that you are on your belly. Then, think about how you can move forward from that position. You cannot get up on your hands and knees and crawl. No, you must find a way to move while being flat on your belly. You won't have done this since you were a very small child. That is the point of the exercise: to make you think and move in that way once again. Therefore, this may bring up all the emotions of that time. If you are not ready for that, it is not for you. You may feel deep sadness, and you may feel the need to cry. There may be many strong emotions you feel as a result of being back in this position.

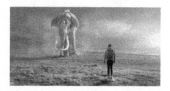

5

TOWERING ABOVE PHYSICAL
PAIN AND ILLNESS

I f you find you are always in pain and have tense muscles or aching bones, this could be the chapter for you. You have become so used to being in pain or muscular tension that you feel like it's almost part of who you are. The good news is that physical somatic therapy (officially called somatics) can help you soothe that pain and get back to feeling yourself. Of course, I must point out that somatic therapy is not for healing just any and every physical injury you have. If you have broken your leg, you still need to see a doctor. You are not going to heal a broken bone through somatic therapy; in fact, you may make things a lot worse. However, if you are affected by chronic muscle and joint pain, then that is where somatic therapy can come in. With its ability to get the body to speak to the brain and vice versa, it is possible to alleviate your pain caused by the twists and stuck muscles to which your body has become accustomed.

Here are a few exercises that should really help you with your mobility and general wellness if you are experiencing chronic pain or tight muscles. You can do all the movements in each step 10 times:

- **1:** Lie on your back with your knees bent and your arms by your sides. Inhale, push your pelvis up slightly, and exhale. Inhale, push your lower back down, and exhale.
- **2:** Lie on your back with legs outstretched and your hands stretched out behind you. You are basically going into a star shape. Pretend you can make your right leg grow longer. Inhale as you imagine doing that, and then exhale and relax. Do the same with your left arm: Imagine it is growing or that someone is pulling your arm to make it longer. Do the same with the left leg and finally with the right arm.
- **3:** Lie on your back with arms outstretched sideways, your knees bent, and then cross one leg over the other. Inhale. Then, move your legs over to the left. Make sure this part is just your legs—everything else will remain central and exhale. Switch legs and do the same, bringing your legs down to the right and back to the center. Then, do the same but with your right arm pointing up and your left hand pointing down. While moving your legs, move your head to the left and vice versa.
- **4:** Get into a sitting position and just rotate your head and torso to the left. Then do the same to the right. Now, do the same but put your right hand on your left shoulder, and after you have rotated, move your head gently back to the center. Then return everything to the center. Do the same for the other side.

SENSORY MOTOR AMNESIA

Sensory motor amnesia (SMA) is a phrase that the pioneer Thomas Hanna, a visionary in the world of somatics, introduced (Warren, 2019). It describes the pattern of physical behavior that your body's muscles carry out without you even thinking about it, which often does you a disservice. For example, day after day, you slouch at your desk over your laptop. Your back muscles become used to this and adapt accordingly so that something bad for you actually becomes normal for your body, and you do nothing to correct it because your body does not tell you to. In fact, quite often, the opposite occurs. Now, sitting up straight becomes painful, and slouching becomes very comfortable. This pattern can then lead to chronic physical pain. In this example, you are likely to end up with severe back pain or maybe even a hump, and you will be forever crouched over, even when standing.

It is easy in the modern world to develop SMA. We are forever slouched over desks, slumped in chairs, and sitting in cars or public transport. We do not move as much as we should, so our body adapts accordingly. It no longer bothers with all that twisting, running, and flexibility you used to need: Our muscles instead focus on what they need to do for slouching and slumping. In turn, muscles can become habitually stuck in unwanted positions, even pulling bones out of place over time.

Another way you can develop SMA is if you have some kind of injury. Then, while your injury heals, it affects how you are moving. This is particularly true if you injure your foot—it affects the way you walk. Then, once your injury has healed, you're still walking in the way you were when you were injured. This is doing you harm, and your body has forgotten how you used to move about normally. Another example would be an injury such as a twisted pelvis.

If you have SMA, you may notice that sometimes, your body is hesitant about its movement; maybe there is a slight shaking or jerking of the affected areas, or there may even be a shudder when your body has let go of some of its tension.

You can do a very simple exercise if you believe you have SMA and would like some confirmation. I advise you that if while doing this exercise you come across pain, take it very slowly and only move within what is acceptable to you; don't try and force anything, as you are only likely to do yourself further damage. It is good to do this exercise slowly to give your brain the chance to comprehend what you are doing. If you do things quickly, the automatic part of your brain will start taking over.

Sit down with your arms down by your sides. Turn your head to the left. You will need to stay looking left throughout the exercise, so make sure your head turn is within your comfort zone and not too painful or stretched. Now, you are going to look up toward the ceiling and move your right shoulder up toward the back of your head. Then, slowly release that position and go back to the position you were in before. You can try this on the other side as well. How did it feel? A bit hesitant or shuddery or shaky? If it was, then you probably do have SMA.

A practice known as pandiculation can help bring about the link between the brain and the muscles and help you to ease your SMA problems.

SOMATIC PANDICULATION

Pandiculation may sound like the most complicated word in the world, but it's really quite a simple concept. Pandiculation involves intentionally (or sometimes, subconsciously) moving muscles to link the movements to our nervous system. The morning stretch and yawn is a perfect example of this. It's a recalibration of our body with our nervous system to further etch movement patterns into our being. We often do this unintentionally and subconsciously when we wake up, but pandiculations can be done on purpose at any time to bring about a myriad of desired results. There are countless somatic pandiculation videos online that target different muscles for different reasons. This act may be more significant than you realize. Bad posture, tight muscles, and unagile movement may become habituated if we don't engage in pandiculation.

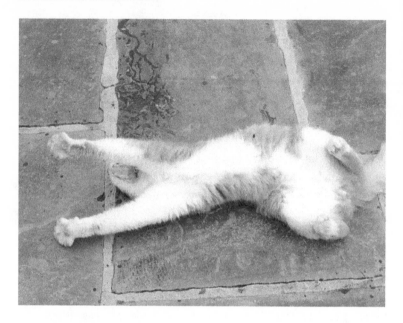

Pandiculation is best explained as the nervous system setting off our internal alarm and saying to the body, "Get ready for some movement!" Humans and any animals with vertebrae tend to automatically perform pandiculation when they wake up or if they have been stationary for a very long while. You probably notice that a baby performs this when they wake up, or you may have seen your pet cat or dog arch their back and stretch out when they have woken up from a doze. All of these are examples of pandiculation. In fact, it is said that animals pandiculate 40 times a day ("Pandiculation—the Safe Alternative to Stretching," 2010). You don't see them all slouched over with bad posture or twisting their ankles just because they had to go and chase a mouse or a stick.

Pandiculation lets our nervous system know the level of tension in our muscles and regulates and resets that muscular tension so we don't end up with muscular pain in the long term. It has been suggested that a fetus can perform pandiculation while in the womb, showing what a primitive and vital action it is (Warren, 2019).

Sadly, with all the bad habits and patterns of physical behavior we so easily get ourselves into in the modern world, automatic pandiculation is just not enough to rid ourselves of all that muscle tension. Sometimes, if our posture is pulled out of alignment, our nervous systems can simply forget to do much pandiculation at all.

Thomas Hanna studied pandiculation in great detail and came to the realization that pandiculation addressed muscle tension and most of the underlying causes of people who had posture issues, movement issues, and chronic pain. He devised some exercises that people could do themselves, rather than relying on automatic pandiculation. He would ensure people were much more equipped to deal with their muscular tensions and free themselves from much of their pain by encouraging voluntary pandiculation. Voluntary pandiculation must be carried out very slowly and intentionally so that the nervous system takes on board what it is being told and updates itself in response (Warren, 2019).

Any pandiculation exercise will require three main aspects:

- **1:** Contract the muscle.
- **2:** Have a slow, intent lengthening of the muscle.
- **3:** Relax as you let your brain and nervous system comprehend what you have just done.

The psoas [**soh**-*uhs*] is an exceptionally important muscle in the human body. Without such muscles, you wouldn't be able to even get yourself out of bed in the morning. That's how important it is. The psoas muscle is also relevant to the way you breathe, so it can have a psychological impact—not just a physical one. Whatever you are doing—running, riding a bike, sitting on the sofa, or dancing— your psoas muscle is required and will be doing work to enable you to do these things. The psoas is so important because it's the muscle that connects your body to your legs. These muscles are otherwise known as the hip flexors. They are extremely vital when it comes to your posture and supporting and regulating your spine. Since the psoas muscle is also connected to the diaphragm, it's prevalent in walking, breathing, and even responding to fear and excitement. If you are under stress, your psoas muscle actually contracts. Essentially, it has a direct impact on your fight-or-flight response. If that stress goes on for long periods, then your psoas muscle is contracted for long periods, leading to a myriad of health issues. That same contraction can happen if you sit down for a long time, run or walk too much, fall and stay asleep in the fetal position, or do a huge amount of sit-ups.

A tight psoas muscle can lead to any number of health issues and complaints, including digestive issues, exhaustion, sexual dysfunction, lower back pain, pelvic pain (which can impact sexual practices and appetite), sciatica (which can cause intolerable pain), a limp, a difference between the length of your legs, curvature in the spine, and a weak core.

You may think that stretching the psoas muscle may be enough, but the psoas muscle takes its instructions from the brain. No matter how much you stretch it, it will be doing what the brain tells it to, and if that is to contract, then contract it will. You could, therefore, end up doing more harm than good by stretching. The best you can achieve is that you may be able to loosen the muscles for a little while after stretching, but soon after, the brain will reset the nervous system, and the psoas muscle will go back to how it was before stretching. Any potential long-term tension can still occur.

I'm going to give you two very simple pandiculation exercises that you can easily complete at home. If you are having trouble with your psoas, these will help you release that tension and trauma and help you open up your life to a world that is free of pain. (Please note: if your psoas doesn't release or re-contracts after pandiculation exercises, then you may be suffering from a twisted sacrum, also known as sacral torsion, a twisted pelvis, or SI joint dysfunction. You'll need to fix a turned sacrum first. I recommend the program "comforting your SI joints" by somatic educator Lawrence Gold.)

- **1:** First, lie on the floor. A flat surface is preferable to a carpet. If you have an exercise mat, that may provide extra comfort. Lie on your back with your knees up and your feet firmly on the floor. Make sure that you can easily slide your foot and leg along the floor (hence, carpet is not such a good surface for this). Put your arms and hands behind your head. Now, take a breath in and arch ever so slightly so that your pelvis moves toward the ceiling and your back contracts; then breathe out and relax.

- Then, when you next breathe out, bring your head and back forward and have your elbows pointing toward your leg. Then, bring one of your legs toward your elbow, then slowly move everything back to where it was: Your head and back to the floor with your elbows and hands behind your head, and your knee and leg back to the floor with your foot planted firmly on the ground.

- Then, do the same with the other side. Take a breath in and arch very slightly, then breathe out and relax; on your next breath out, move your other knee toward your elbows and then slowly move everything back to where it was before.

- Next, do the same exercise, but when you put your foot back on the floor, slide your leg and foot all the way along the ground and flex your toes. Breathe in and out as you require. You can also slightly vary so that when you next bring your leg up and put it down, it comes up more naturally so that your leg and foot are curved outward rather than straight. You can repeat the exercise several times with both legs. It will be interesting to see if you notice any difference between each side; maybe one side feels less tight than the other. Whatever you notice, after doing these exercises for a while, you will see that your psoas is not as tight, and you have managed to release some of that tension out of your body.

- **2:** Do the same exercise, but this time, keep your arms by your side when you lift your knee up. Then, when you slide your leg out this time, bring your arm over your head from your side—as if when you swim, you are doing the backstroke. Do one stroke, put your arm over your head, and relax. Go back into position, repeat, and then do the same with the other side of your body. This exercise will help with the muscles toward the upper part of your back; if your psoas is tight, you should feel that along the side of your body.

There are also some straightforward exercises you can do to ensure all the various muscle groups undergo pandiculation.

- This one will help work your biceps. You can do this standing up or sitting down. Just bring your forearm toward you slowly as though you were lifting a dumbbell, and then let it slowly go back to its position and relax. If you need to, you can lightly place your first two fingers of your other hand onto your arm just to put a tiny bit of resistance there, and that helps your brain and nervous system work out what is going on and not cause any SMA possibilities.
- I definitely have a problem constantly pushing my head out in front of me, particularly when hunched over my laptop. An exercise to help remedy that is the following: Kneel down, arch slowly, slowly pull your belly and head back, and then relax. Again, if you need a little bit of resistance to help, you can place one hand under your chest and one hand on your belly. Your spine and the

front of your body should feel more in harmony after doing this exercise. Rather than being hunched over with your head forward, you should be able to sit up straight with your head sitting nicely on the top of your body where it is meant to be.

These exercises should really help you in the long term in a way that stretching simply cannot. You are performing pandiculation on your muscles that will work wonders for you. With some luck, the days of never-ending pain, inflexibility, or struggle in your movement will be gone. All helped with something that you can easily do at home for free.

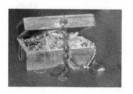

6

A TREASURE TROVE OF SOMATIC
PRACTICES

In this chapter, I am going to outline some of the most powerful somatic practices. It really is a treasure trove of a chapter. All these years have been like digging for diamonds or panning for gold without any luck—until now. You are going to find that treasure you needed—your pot of gold at the end of the rainbow. These are easy-to-follow practices that you can do in your own time and space. They do not require special equipment or great expense to be able to take part in them. Best of all, there is genuine scientific evidence backing up these practices, so I know they work; soon, you will, too.

POLYVAGAL THEORY AND THE VAGUS NERVE

The polyvagal theory was developed by Stephen Porges and helps us to better understand our nervous system. It came out of his studying of the vagus nerve. The vagus nerve is involved in the calming element of the nervous system. This balances out with the active element, so if there is more calming occurring, then less activity is needed. If more activity is occurring, then less calming is needed. Polyvagal theory describes a third element, what Porges labeled as the "Social Engagement System"—a combination of both the active and the calming aspects (Wagner, 2016).

As the name suggests, it is the social engagement aspect that assists us in working our way through relationships and to better cope with any conflict that may arise.

The nervous system has two main elements when it comes to feeling like we are in grave danger: the element that deals with our fight-or-flight response and the part that deals with shutting down completely (think back to the "flop" method of dealing with danger). In order for the social engagement system to become engaged, there has to be a sense of being safe.

It is the vagus nerve that helps calm the body, and it has two main aspects to it, which behave in very different ways. The shutting down aspect occurs through one part of the vagus nerve. When this shutdown occurs, a person will usually feel very tired and maybe quite giddy—rather like if you had the flu. This can affect a person's heart, lungs, diaphragm, and digestive system.

The other part of the vagus nerve affects things above the diaphragm. This is the part that services the social engagement system. This part of the nerve helps to control our nervous system. For example, if you are letting someone rock climb, you let the rope down slowly for them to work their way down safely; you don't let the rope go all at once. That is kind of what the vagus nerve is doing here: keeping your nervous system regulated and stopping it from becoming hyperactive. Whereas the fight-or-flight response can take seconds to take place and recovery can take anywhere from 10 to 20 minutes, the vagus nerve's response to calm takes mere milliseconds. Therefore, we should be able to calm our responses in the same way you let down the rope slowly for a rock climber to control their ascent down the face of a cliff.

A good example of social engagement in action is if you go down to your local park and observe the dogs. Some dogs will be aggressive toward other dogs or will run away, and their owners have to chase after them—these are the dogs in fight-or-flight mode. But if you see the dogs happily playing, wagging their tails, wanting a stick or ball to be thrown, and jumping up in a friendly way at their owners, these are the dogs who feel in a safe space and are employing the social engagement system.

If a person has trauma that they have not managed to release, then they can find themselves forever in a world of fight or flight; instead of happily going about their daily activities with their social engagement system fully in tune, everything becomes a task of dread and fear.

The vagus nerve actually impacts the middle ear, which can help us focus on human voices and remove all the unnecessary background noise. It also impacts our ability to make facial expressions —another essential for communication. Finally, it also impacts our vocal cords and the noises we may make to each other—again, to communicate in a calming manner. It is the longest nerve in the body, and if you are wondering how it got its name, it's because, in Latin, *vagus* means "wandering." You know it's a long nerve when it's named the "wandering" nerve.

Ultimately, if we can find ways to reset that vagal nerve or exercise it so that we feel happy, safe, secure, and playful, then life can be so much better for us.

EXERCISE #1

First is a really simple exercise. Start by sitting up and moving your head slowly to the left, back to the center, and then to the right. Is there any difference between each side? Do you find it more difficult to move your head to one side compared to the other? When I first discovered this exercise, I found it slightly more difficult to move my head to the right side compared to the left side. After this, lie down on your back with your knees up and your feet firmly on the floor. Once you become experienced at this exercise, you can do it sitting up or even standing up, but you should lie down for it for the first few times. Place your hands behind your head, with your fingers interlocked and your elbows pointing out so that you are holding your head in your hands. Then, move your eyes to the right—not your head: just your eyes. Use your hands to support your head so you don't move it. You only move your eyes. Hold your eyes in that position for 30 seconds. Then, relax and let your eyes come back to the middle. If you notice that you may need to take a breath or have the urge to swallow, those are vagus nerve responses and signs that the exercise is working.

Now, do the other side: Move your eyes to the left, with your head not moving and staying central, and hold your eyes there for 30 seconds. Then, relax and let your eyes come back to the middle. Take a moment, then return to your sitting position and move your head side to side to see if your mobility has improved. By the way, 30 seconds is the minimum time to hold your eyes in position. If you are not getting any of the signs, like a deep breath or swallowing, you can hold your eyes in position for 60 seconds or more. When I first discovered this exercise, I found it slightly more difficult to turn my head to the right side. Once I had done the exercise, then I found I could move my head without restriction equally on both sides. This exercise works.

EXERCISE #2

The second exercise you can do is to just sit down. Whether that be on the floor or in a chair—as long as you are comfortable, that is the main thing. Place your right hand on the top of your head, and then tip your head to the right. Move your eyes and your eyes only. Hold that position for 30 seconds. You can relax after that and resume your normal sitting position. Now, you will do the same but for the other side. Put your left hand on your head, and tip your head to the left. Move your eyes up and to the right. Hold the position for 30 seconds. Again, you can hold the position longer if you are not feeling any effect.

EXERCISE #3

For the third exercise, again, be in a sitting position, take your right hand, and put it on top of your head, tipping your head to the right. However, this time, take your left hand and reach around to clutch your right side. Then, move your head to the right side, and use your left hand to pull your side. Again, move your eyes only, up and to the left, and hold the position for 30 seconds. Then, release yourself from the position and relax. You should notice yourself feeling a bit calmer having performed that exercise. Do the other side: left hand on top of your head and tip your head to the left. Use your right hand to reach around to your left side and pull your side. Then, move your eyes up and to the right side and hold the position for 30 seconds. Once again, release yourself from that position and relax.

EXERCISE #4

For this next exercise, you need to find somewhere comfortable to lie down. If you have an exercise or yoga mat, that is probably best. I found lying face down on a carpeted floor isn't much fun, as it usually just reminds me I need to get the vacuum cleaner out! Once ready, you are going to prop yourself up on your elbows, hands pointing out in front of you and flat on the floor. Then, you are going to turn to your left and look over your shoulder. As per usual, hold the position for 30 seconds. Release that position and relax; lie face down if you want to for a few moments. Now, do the same thing but look over your right shoulder this time. Hold the position for 30 seconds, then release yourself from the position and relax. As you are using your neck muscles in this exercise, it can be really good for those who have tension in that area and, as a result, suffer from headaches and migraines. Do this exercise, and you should release some of the tension and be able to get some relief from the pain.

Believe it or not, breathing can also have an impact on your vagus nerve and your vagus nerve on your breathing. That is something known as "vagal tone," which basically represents your vagus nerve activity (Fallis, 2021). The higher your vagal tone is, the easier you will find it to return to a relaxed state after a moment of stress. If we can find a way to activate our vagal nerve and increase our vagal tone, then we should feel less stressed, less anxious, and generally happier. A 2010 study found that those with a high vagal tone were generally positive in their feelings and had good physical health (Kok et al., 2013). There have even been studies that suggest that if mothers are anxious and stressed during pregnancy (giving them a low vagal tone), this actually gets passed on to the baby when it is born, and the baby also shares a low vagal tone (Field & Diego, 2008). There has even been a device that can be planted in you that will activate your vagus nerve every so often, but that is an extreme way to go. Deep and slow breathwork can activate your vagus nerve and increase your vagal tone.

Therefore, at this point, it would be good to give you some breathing exercises to activate your vagal tone. These exercises all have different purposes. This first one is to enable you to relax.

BREATHING EXERCISE #1

You can start by sitting down and putting your arms around your rib cage and your belly, or you can use a pillow to put in front of you and use that. You are basically putting yourself into a hug position. Then, breathe in until you have a full feeling and hold for four seconds; after, breathe out for longer than you breathed in and hold for six seconds. You can "hug" yourself a little harder when you breathe out if you like because that is what is activating the vagus nerve. You can then transpose this exercise to the floor to make it even more relaxing. You can lie on your back or your front. If you are on your back with your knees up and feet firmly on the floor, you can put pressure on your belly and your chest with your hands.

If you are lying on your front, you can lie down stretched out, and you can put a pillow or cushion under your belly or chest to add some pressure.

You then breathe in for six seconds and hold it for four. See if you can feel your heartbeat rhythm and use that as your count of four. Breathe out for eight seconds and then hold that for four seconds; keep repeating. If you feel you can increase the time you exhale, try to do that. It is that exhaling length that really alerts the vagus nerve and gets you to a place of relaxation. One last thing you can do to relax even further is to lie on your back with your knees up and feet firmly on the floor. Place something under your buttocks and lower back. This is to ensure your pelvis is raised up higher than your head. When there is too much blood flowing toward your head, this immediately alerts the vagus nerve and starts slowing down your heart rate and relaxing you. Breathe in until you feel full. Swallow and breathe out for longer than you breathed in. After, just take a momentary pause until you feel the need to breathe in again. Then, breathe in until you feel full. Swallow and breathe out for longer than you breathed in. Pause until you need to breathe in again. Keep repeating. This should see you enter a state of deep relaxation and calmness.

BREATHING EXERCISE #2

This next exercise is a nice and easy one you can use whenever you want, which will activate the vagus nerve. Vocalizing sounds can be really beneficial—that's why singing usually feels so good to you. The first sound to make is an "mmm" sound. Take a deep breath—with your belly, not a shallow breath with your chest—and when you breathe out, make that "mmm" sound for as long as you can. Take a deep breath again, and when you breathe out, make an "ahhh" sound this time. Take a deep breath, and when you breathe, make an "ooh" sound. Finally, take a deep breath and make all three sounds in a row until you run out of breath: "mmm, ahhh, ooh."

Making these sounds is a really good way to activate that vagus nerve for those times when you are feeling stressed.

GUIDED MEDITATION

I'm now going to provide you with a guided meditation for vagus nerve stimulation. As with all the vagus nerve exercises, this should help you relax, feel calm, and release any tension. For this, you need to make sure you are sitting up comfortably.

- **1:** Make sure you breathe from your belly and diaphragm, and you're not shallow breathing from your chest.
  Breathe in for six seconds and hold for four seconds.
- **2:** Breathe out for eight seconds and hold for four seconds.
- **3:** Keep repeating.
- **4:** The most important thing to remember is that your breathing out should last longer than your breathing in. Even if you become relaxed enough to stop counting, you need to make sure the exhale is longer than the inhale. That long breath out stimulates the vagus nerve, leaves you feeling calm, and releases any tension.
- **5:** You can stop your breathing, become aware of your whole body again, and when you feel ready, you can open your eyes.

PENDULATION

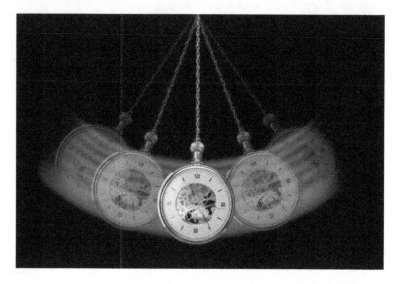

Pendulation is a term devised by the king of somatic experiencing, Peter Levine. As you could probably guess from its name, it describes something similar to a pendulum, but what is swinging, in this case, are your feelings, emotions, and nervous system. You are swinging between that state, which is fear and fight or flight, and the calm and relaxed state where your vagus nerve is stimulated and your vagal tone is high. If a person can learn to move between those two states, then when a person gets into a state of anxiety, stress, and feels tense or in pain, they can learn to swing to the other state and stand a chance of becoming more relaxed, peaceful, and at ease. Of course, it is never quite that simple. Sometimes, all you can do is move to a less painful or less anxious state, but that is still a better place to be than where you started. It also means that you can do so in small pieces when you go to those dark and worrying places. You are in control, so you don't have to go through everything all at once. You can deal with it and then get back to your safe and secure space. After all, how can you really know what feeling happy is unless you have felt sad as well? How can you know what calm means without feeling stressed? Both states have to exist, and we have to understand and learn to appreciate the negative as well as the positive.

Peter Levine compares it to contraction and expansion: The basic rhythm of life is contraction and expansion. However, when a person becomes traumatized, the rhythm becomes contraction and nothing else. Through pendulation, the contraction can slowly be opened up to an expansion. Then, there will still be a contraction— the rhythm of life—but there will be an expansion until the person becomes able to tolerate the contraction, knowing that a bigger expansion is coming. Those who are happy with life and living it to the fullest learn to respect and appreciate the contraction, knowing it leads to expansion when they are calm and open (Somatic Experiencing International, 2019).

In a moment, we'll look at a pendulation exercise. This first exercise is particularly useful if you are in pain or feel tension in one specific part of your body.

PENDULATION EXERCISE

For this exercise, you are going to think about two places on your body. First, think about the part of your body that is in pain. We have to acknowledge the pain in the body before we think about anything else. I often find my upper back can be quite painful if I haven't been sitting properly at my desk, so for this exercise, I may focus on that and acknowledge the pain there, but, at the same time, maybe give it a rub and let it know I care for it. Then, think of a part of your body that isn't in pain and doesn't give you any problems. Maybe it's your hair; perhaps it's your big toe. Whatever it is, think of that and how good it is, how it's free of pain, and how it helps you achieve what you want. Then, switch between the two —thinking about the pain and then the good part of your body. Going back and forth is the pendulation aspect. Contract pain, and expand part of your body that is good. As I say, this exercise is good if you have a particular part of your body in pain or if you are anxious and that has manifested as a physical symptom. You focus on that—maybe it's an upset stomach, a headache, or maybe your arms feel itchy. Switch to thinking about a part of your body that is not impacted and switch between the two. Your anxiety should gradually ease as you acknowledge the anxiety but also acknowledge a part of your body that is working well for you. You may want to slow down your breathing as you do the switching to help give you that extra level and activation of your vagus nerve to help calm you down.

SOMATIC TITRATION

Titration may have a complex-sounding name, but it is not a complex concept to understand. It is the process of slowly tackling the trauma. If a person were to consider their trauma all at once, it would be too much, and they would become overwhelmed. It is the process of slowly remembering and becoming comfortable with your trauma. It is not just the slowing down of the trauma but slowing down to take time to appreciate how your body is feeling, the sensations you are picking up, and the world around you. It could be said that pendulation uses titration because you don't just focus on the part that hurts: You focus on that for a bit, then on something that isn't hurting and come back. You are slowly thinking about the trauma. You don't just focus on the part that hurts forever until it completely overwhelms you.

The name "titration" comes from a chemistry term that describes slowly dripping potentially dangerous chemicals into a beaker so that the chemical change—turning these chemicals into a harmless substance—occurs safely. The unsafe option would be to put the chemicals in all at once, causing an explosion.

COGNITIVE BEHAVIORAL THERAPY

Cognitive behavioral therapy (CBT) is a type of therapy specifically aimed at those who may have mental health difficulties. It is based on the theory that people have ways of thinking that are not beneficial to them, and these unhelpful ways of thinking become a habit or a pattern of behavior. By teaching people more helpful ways of thinking about things, they may be able to cope much better with their anxiety, depression, or whatever issues they may be having and maybe even relieve themselves of those issues.

As CBT involves changing the way you think about things and your thinking behavior patterns, it will usually include getting a person to realize where their thinking is exaggerated or less moderated. Try to get the person to recognize the reality of that situation and change their thinking accordingly. It may provide certain issue resolution skills to assist the person with particularly complex situations. It may also include providing the person with confidence in themselves and their instincts.

I have had close family members go through CBT. While I realize and appreciate its ability to get a person to cope better with what they are going through—providing them with the tool kit to apply whenever they feel things are spiraling out of control—It doesn't always address the root cause of the problem. It often overlooks the actual cause of their depression or anxiety.

However, I can't deny the evidence that exists to support the view that CBT can make a big difference in someone else's life and help them contain and control the difficulties they are going through. A study of analysis from controlled trials concluded that CBT was effective when dealing with major depression, though its effect was not huge (Lynch et al., 2009). A similar study dealing with previous data concluded that CBT effectively dealt with many cases of depression, anxiety, panic disorders, social phobias, and PTSD (Butler at al., 2006). As there is empirical evidence to support the effectiveness of CBT, this has led to its use as an official treatment for those with mental health issues.

You may think CBT is something you have to do in conjunction with a therapist, but, in fact, what the therapist does is give you the tools to use yourself in your daily life to help combat your worst thoughts and feelings. Overall, it is possible to do exercises yourself. I will outline an excellent, simple CBT exercise to follow here. This one is particularly for those who may often find themselves depressed or possibly anxious.

CBT EXERCISE #1

First, write down the negative thoughts you have in your head. Maybe it's, "No one likes me," "I am useless," or whatever destabilizing thought it could be. Then, write down the opposite positive possibility: "I am likable" or, "I do have use." Initially, it can be very hard to accept the second statement. Still, over time, the more you repeat the exercise and feel comfortable with yourself, the more you will start to accept the second statement as fact.

CBT EXERCISE #2

Another exercise you can engage in is if you naturally think negatively about something. Try to ignore that negative thought and concentrate on five positive things instead. Imagine you don't like a room because you hate the carpet; try to think of the five positive things about the room—you like the large windows, you like the large doors, you like the paintings on the wall, you like the roundness of the table, and you like the light coming through when it's sunny outside. Try to think of five good things about whatever you are feeling negative about. If you can find someone else to do this with, then even better: You will be able to work off each other and get some enthusiasm for finding positives.

ENERGY PSYCHOLOGY

What is energy psychology? Well, David Feinstein, an early advocate of energy psychology, described it nicely as "acupuncture without the needles" ("Energy Psychology," 2017). Although that simplifies it somewhat, this is an accurate description. Energy psychology involves tapping various points on your body, which will then send messages back to the brain to regulate your emotions and feelings and help calm and relax you. Usually, the tapping is carried out in tandem with becoming aware of the body and the feelings, thoughts, and behaviors that may need to change. Someone having this type of therapy may be asked to remember a traumatic event while the body tapping is carried out.

If trauma is trapped in the body, then using tapping can be the way to release that trauma and bring relief and peace to a person. There are various types and techniques of energy psychology that are practiced. ("Energy Psychology," 2017) These include :

- **Thought Field Therapy (TFT):** This type of therapy requires body tapping to occur in a very specific order. A person will be required to recall a traumatic event, and then the tapping will occur in the required sequence. This form of therapy was developed by Dr. Roger Callaghan, who claimed to have formed algorithms that pertained to the correct order in which to perform the tapping.
- **Tapas Acupressure Technique (TAT):** The word tapas makes me hungry. However, this technique has nothing to do with bite-sized Spanish food. The title of this technique takes its name from the man who invented it: Tapas Fleming. This technique requires someone to use their fingers to apply pressure to areas around the eyes, above the nose, and on the back of the head. The person may then need to focus on images that

have caused them distress in the past and to then focus on more positive images. They might then focus on what they believe may have caused their issues and then focus on healing and forgiveness.

- **Emotional Freedom Techniques (EFT):** This technique is not unlike the others. It requires a person to recall a traumatic event and then for tapping to occur on 12 points on the body in a specific order while the person declares affirmations. This technique was developed by Gary Craig and is a variant of "Thought Field Therapy."

These may sound like the kind of practices you would need a therapist to perform on you, but they are all techniques that can be self-taught and carried out by an individual. Like all the therapies and techniques in this book, it is easy to find time to incorporate them into your daily routine.

As with many new therapies, the jury is still out on genuine scientific evidence to prove the true value of energy psychology, but research is emerging that suggests it can positively impact those who have trauma, anxiety, and stress. Feinstein carried out research on all the studies that had taken place and concluded that energy psychology did make a valuable difference when treating those with emotional and psychological issues (Feinstein, 2012). Of course, Feinstein is a big advocate of energy psychology, so to be fair, one has to take what he says with a pinch of salt. However, he references many independent studies from all over the world, so one can also conclude that there must be something in it if so many people are noticing the positive difference it can make. Personally, I am a huge advocate of EFT tapping and make sure to practice at least three sessions per day. I have noticed a profound positive difference in my anxiety, OCD, and countless other traits.

ENERGY PSYCHOLOGY EXERCISE #1

Ready to try an energy psychology exercise? Let's go for it. First, make sure you are sitting somewhere comfortably. Now, find an area on the left side of your chest or just above that maybe feels a little sore or tight. Give that a little rub using your fingers—make circles with your fingers over that area—and then you can say some affirmations at the same time. Maybe try saying, "I love, respect, and cherish myself—even my flaws." You can continue to say that as you rub the sore area. Then, breathe in deeply and breathe out very slowly. Pause momentarily and consider how you feel and how your body feels afterward.

ENERGY PSYCHOLOGY EXERCISE #2

For this next exercise, you need to cross your left ankle over your right and put your arms in the air out in front of you—facing outward so that your thumbs are facing down. Do the opposite with your hands as you did with your ankles. Clasp your hands together so your fingers are interlocking, and roll your hands in. Then, put your hands on your chest in the most comfortable way possible. Now, inhale through your nose and exhale through your mouth. Do this five times. You can relax after that. Uncross everything and pause again to consider how you and your body feels. Then, do the same exercise, but this time, put your right ankle over your left and your left hand over your right. Turn your hands and arms in again, and, as with last time, inhale through your nose and exhale through your mouth five times. Once you've done that, relax and uncross everything. Take a moment to think about how you feel and how your body feels. Finally, just to round things off, put your five fingers from both hands together and up, so you are making a kind of pyramid with your hands. Feel present and aware in that moment. Breathe deeply using your belly and not your chest. After a few breaths, relax and think about how you feel again.

ENERGY PSYCHOLOGY EXERCISE #3

Once you feel confident with the ankle and hand-crossing exercise, there is a slightly more complex version you may want to take on. This involves looking up toward the ceiling or sky when inhaling and looking down at the floor when exhaling. Then, just to make things even more complicated for you, move your tongue to the roof of your mouth when inhaling, and move your tongue to the bottom of the mouth when exhaling. There is quite a bit to remember with this version of the exercise, so start with the simple exercise, and once you have that down to a tee, perhaps you can move on to this more complex version and see how it goes. After, relax and uncross everything. Once again, make the pyramid shape with your hands and take some time to be in the moment and aware of how your body feels. As you can see, there's no tapping your forehead or having to lie down and get in difficult positions. This is something you can easily fit into your day—maybe when you wake up or before you go to sleep. Any moment you get a few minutes to yourself, aim to do these exercises.

SENSORIMOTOR PSYCHOTHERAPY

The people responsible for naming therapies love giving difficult names to them, don't they? Sensorimotor psychotherapy comes from the sensory motor, which we had previously encountered in this book when discussing sensory motor amnesia. This type of psychotherapy, like most in the somatic therapy arena, concentrates on the body to unlock and release trapped trauma.

Pat Ogden first came to develop this kind of therapy after working in a psychiatric hospital and realizing that patients there never linked their physical ailments with their mental health issues. She noticed that those who attended therapy tended to relive and trigger their traumatic experiences, and it didn't really help heal them. Ogden set about rectifying this situation by combining elements of psychotherapy with elements of somatic therapy—something that would emphasize the link between the body and the mind: not ignore it. Ogden joined together with Ron Kurtz, and together, they formed a training institute known as the Sensorimotor Psychotherapy Institute (Sensorimotor Psychotherapy, 2015).

Like most somatic therapies, sensorimotor psychotherapy believes that trauma can become trapped in the body if not dealt with fully at the time, so it can result in both physical and mental problems. It tries to close off that trauma in a safe space. It does not necessarily believe that a trauma's exact specifics need to be recalled to effectively release it.

Although how sensorimotor psychotherapy is applied can vary depending on the practitioners and the issues it is addressing, there are three main elements that need to be focused on:

- **1: Creating a Safe Space:** Doing this enables a person to feel comfortable and allows them to really be aware of their body, their feelings and sensations, their movements, and their breathing patterns. Having a place where the person feels protected really helps them be aware of their body and what it is feeling both in the moment and when related to past experiences.

- **2:** As a person recalls their traumatic experience, both **what they feel** and **where they feel** it is noted. For example, if a person says they feel anxious, where do they feel it? Does their stomach feel tied in knots? Is it causing a headache? Do they feel the need to scratch their skin? This can then help with trying to reimagine any traumatic events by incorporating those bodily feelings.

- **3:** The person needs to **complete the required action** that will allow the trauma to be released. This should give the person a sense of satisfaction as they finally do what needs to be done and put the trauma to one side. The person should be able to find that calm and peace that exists when trauma is finally put into the past and stays there.

Sensorimotor psychotherapy aims to give people the ability to control their reactions to traumatic events and an awareness of how trauma can impact the body—not just the mind. It also looks to provide the tools to tell the difference between the past and the present. It helps with being able to consider thoughts and feelings —both in mind and in the body—rather than becoming over-whelmed by a traumatic event.

There is still not much research on the effectiveness of sensori-motor psychotherapy. However, one study was carried out on ten women with a history of child abuse. They took part in 20 weekly group therapy sessions based on sensorimotor psychotherapy. The study concluded that there had been significant improvements in awareness of bodies, disassociation, and acceptance of peace and calm (Langmuir et al., 2012).

One aspect often employed in sensorimotor psychotherapy is grounding. When you feel like you've lost your footing in the world and are unsteady both mentally and physically, grounding is required. Grounding exercises are described as being able to firmly plant your feet on the ground and taking the time to be aware of your body and everything around you. Here are a few elementary grounding exercises you can practice anywhere:

- There are a few variations you can do. You can place a hand on your forehead and a hand on your heart, a hand on your forehead and your belly, or a hand on your heart and a hand on your belly. Pick your combination, or give them all a go. Once you are in position, apply a tiny bit of pressure with your hands and then breathe deeply.
- Rub your hands together, specifically the palms. Think of

it almost like you had a stick between them, and you needed to create fire. Once your palms have warmed up from the friction, place them over your eyes, apply a tiny little bit of pressure, and breathe deeply.

- Cross your arms over and grab your upper arms, so your left hand will be on your right upper arm, for instance. Squeeze gently and continue to do that all the way down your arms and back up again.

- Put your right hand on the left side of your chest and stroke (like you would a cat) down from your shoulder to your heart. I must say I find that one particularly comforting, but then they say stroking a cat can be therapeutic; maybe it's the stroking that I find comfort in.

- Put one foot on top of the other and apply a little pressure. Change over your feet and do the same.

These are just some simple exercises that you can do at home. Generally, sensorimotor psychotherapy is a form of therapy that needs a therapist to guide you and interpret for you more than some other therapies. Still, it is nothing you cannot teach yourself. With the grounding exercises, I have already given you a head start on activities you can easily practice at home.

GESTALT THERAPY

Gestalt therapy is about concentrating on what is happening right now and not basing the present on what may have occurred in the past. Those undergoing gestalt therapy are asked to reimagine those past experiences. Through the various techniques and tools, they become aware of how their own thought patterns and behaviors are negatively impacting their life. If they can change those ways, they can find a fulfilling life.

The word "gestalt" can mean whole, and the psychotherapist

who developed this type of therapy, Fritz Perls, was very much a believer in people being treated as a whole—mind, body, and soul/spirit. He also believed people could only truly be understood when they viewed things through their own eyes, not by mentally going back to the past and staying there, but by bringing the past into the present. Gestalt therapy advocates that it is no good just talking about how a person feels in the past but by reenacting those feelings in the present. If one fails to bring out feelings in the present, this can lead to mental and physical health problems. Peris was a firm believer that we were not put on this earth to try and live up to other people's expectations, and, equally, other people are not obliged to live up to ours (Clarke, 2021). By providing people the ability to become self-aware, they will appreciate the connection between mind and body and find much better ways to deal with all the bows and arrows everyday life can sling at you.

Does it work, though? Well, a study carried out in Hong Kong regarding anxious parents found that after four weeks of gestalt therapy, the parents had lower anxiety levels, were less willing to avoid inner experiences, were kinder to themselves, and demonstrated more mindfulness compared to those that did not go through the therapy (Leung & Khor, 2017). A study carried out on women with depression found that the depression was reduced effectively using gestalt therapy (Heidari et al., 2017). Why these studies seem to concentrate on women, I'm not sure. Still, a study conducted on divorced women concluded after 12 sessions of gestalt therapy, the women showed much more self-belief in their abilities (Saadati & Lashani, 2013).

I would say that gestalt therapy is a form of therapy that is best practiced with a therapist rather than alone. However, there are simple and straightforward gestalt therapy exercises you can do at home if you want to explore this area.

GESTALT THERAPY EXERCISE #1

This exercise is known as a body scan meditation, and it helps us connect with our bodies—an essential part of gestalt therapy and somatic healing therapy. Make sure you find a comfortable and quiet place to lie down. Close your eyes and become aware of your breath, how the air is coming in and out of the body, and how your belly rises and comes down. Take a few minutes to focus on how you are breathing and what your body is doing. After those few minutes, start to focus instead on the toes of your left foot, and imagine your breath rushing all down your body, down your leg, and into those toes. Concentrate on any feelings you may have in your toes, and stay with those feelings—be curious about them. Now, move your focus along your foot—from your toes down to the heel and ankle of your foot. Take your time in moving down. Each time, refocus on that part of the foot and imagine your breath flowing down to that part of your body and what your body feels as a result.

Move through your whole leg right up to your pelvis, doing the same thing. Then do the same with your other leg. Now, focus on your belly and lower back, then through your upper back and chest, and up the rest of your body until you reach your shoulders. After that, focus on the fingers of both hands simultaneously, and move up both your arms until, again, you reach the shoulders. Now, shift your focus to your head, moving up through your neck, chin, mouth, nose, eyes, and everything else, over the back of your head, and finish at the top of your head. Now, switch your focus to the whole of your body, and feel your breath come in through the top of your head and go out through the tips of your toes. Then, feel it come in through your toes and out the top of your head; keep doing this for a few minutes. Then, slowly become aware of your belly rising and falling with each breath again. Begin to move some of your body, such as your hands and feet, and when you feel you are ready, slowly open your eyes. You may want to remain lying down for a while before you finally get up off the ground and start moving around again. You can take the opportunity to note down any particularly strong feelings you had during the meditation or comparisons on how you felt before and after.

FOCUSING THERAPY

Focusing is exactly what it sounds like. You focus on yourself and learn to hear those innermost feelings that your body is trying to tell you. Focusing can be practiced by anyone who has learned the procedures. It can be used as often or little as the person doing the focusing desires. The person doing the focusing is the one that is in control of what goes on.

Focusing was first developed by Eugene Gendlin in the 1950s when he researched what in particular made psychotherapy beneficial to people. He discovered that those that seemingly got the most out of psychotherapy were people who had feelings that were not easily explainable. Still, such people were able to put descriptions or images to these feelings. This resulted in people finding what had yet to be discovered, which allowed the psychotherapy to continue moving forward. Gendlin also noted that this was normally accompanied by a sigh or deep breath from the person, which signified a release of some kind. For those in somatic healing, they may well say it is trauma that is being released (Jordan, 2016).

Gendlin came up with focusing to help those who could not so easily access the ability to excavate these nameless feelings so deeply hidden. Initially, he wrote how focusing consisted of six main steps:

- **1:** Make a space.
- **2:** Find those unknown inner feelings—which Gendlin described as a "felt sense."
- **3:** Find a description or title for your "felt sense."
- **4:** Repeat those titles or descriptions to ensure they correctly match the "felt sense."

- **5:** Try asking: This is where the person focusing will ask themselves questions that can't simply be answered with a "yes" or "no," such as, "What was so difficult about that? Why can't you move past that? What was so lovely about that?"
- **6:** Have a release in your body, which Gendlin termed a "felt shift." It is obviously very beneficial to the person doing the focusing if they do experience a "felt shift," but it is not essential. Focusing is an ongoing process, so where the person doing the focusing may start out and where they may end up can be two very different places (Jordan, 2016).

A study of 87 people found that focusing may be effective in providing support to those who have undergone severe trauma (Zweircan & Joseph, 2018). Some would say the evidence is in Gendlin's own research when he developed the idea of focusing.

Now let's walk through the six steps that Gendlin identified in the form of an exercise, and you can see whether focusing is something you think can make a difference in your life. This exercise can take up to 20 or 30 minutes, so you need to clear some space in your itinerary. Instead of watching a TV show in which you already know what is going to happen, perhaps you can do this exercise instead. You can either lie down on a bed (perhaps do this when you first wake up or before you sleep) or on the ground. You can also sit in a chair with your feet firmly on the ground if you prefer.

- **1:** The first step is to clear the space so that we can do a quick relaxation exercise. Get yourself comfortable and take a deep breath. Notice the weight of your body either on the floor, bed, or chair. Make sure any clothing that may be too tight is loosened, and close your eyes. Breathe in and out, and notice your breath as you are doing this. Do this several times and just be aware of your breathing. Take note of anywhere in your body where there is tension. Picture that tension as a river of water that is running through your body and out your fingers and toes. Continue to breathe, letting that tension run off your fingers and toes. Now, find a place within your body where it feels peaceful.

- **2:** Slowly, move to the next exercise and find that "felt sense." Keep your eyes closed and think about the center of your body. Try to remember an experience in the past week that was of concern or difficulty for you. Think about that experience and try to form an image of it in your mind. Try to put to one side all the thoughts you have had about it and search for that "felt sense"—that feeling you had when that experience occurred and not how you felt about it after. Put aside your thoughts and just try to get the feeling of that experience in you.

- **3:** Now you need to find a title or description or image for that "felt sense." Keep your eyes closed, keep breathing, and see if any words or images come to mind.

- **4:** Repeat that word or image and see if it resonates with you. See if it truly does match that "felt sense" you had in the center of your body about your experience. Keep checking one against the other. You'll know when you have it right, as you'll feel your body be in agreement with you.

- **5:** What do you find you are asking yourself? It depends on each experience what kind of questions may crop up, but maybe you are asking yourself things like, "What is so difficult about this experience for me?" Between each question, you should wait a minute or so to determine what your "felt sense" is telling you. Then, see what words or images come to you to label that feeling. Now, try to get your body to feel what it would be like if that situation or experience you have been pondering was actually all okay. Take a minute or so to feel that. Then, ask yourself, "What is it that's stopping the experience from becoming okay?" Don't answer from your mind. I must say I always find this one difficult to resist but do try. You need to feel it in your body again. As with the other points, this may take a minute or so for something to come to light. Once again, listen to that "felt sense'" in your body and come up with a word or image that can represent what it is that's stopping the experience from being okay. Finally, try to see if you can come up with what might be able to get you from the negative experience to it becoming positive or at least a lot more bearable. Again, don't answer with your mind: Let your body do the talking. Here, you can do some more asking. "Does it feel right to do that?" If your "felt sense" is saying no, then you need to reconsider; if your "felt sense" is saying, "Yes, that's right," then you can stop there.

Hopefully, at the end of that, you feel you have some kind of answer to your problem. Even if not, solutions can crop up later. For the moment, take some time to pause and just appreciate yourself. Appreciate the "thinking" your body has done in connection with the issue you are having.

Then, when you feel ready to do so, open your eyes and start to become aware of the room and everything around you. If you were lucky, you might well have had that release of tension at the end of the fifth step. If you didn't, that's okay. As I stated before, that is not the whole point of focusing. The main point is getting to know your body and understanding and listening to it so that you truly know what you are feeling and what's the best way forward to resolve your issues.

PSYCHODRAMA THERAPY

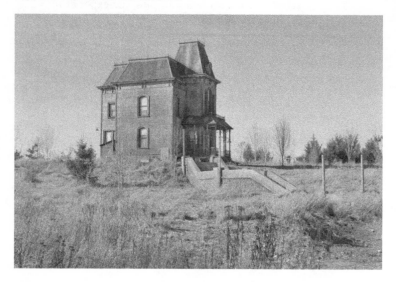

Don't worry. This doesn't involve Anthony Perkins in a wig from *Psycho* or anything like that. Psychodrama Therapy is a form of therapy that requires a person to engage in actions in order to resolve their problems. This can include role-playing and group therapy.

Psychodrama came into fruition in the early 1900s thanks to the psychiatrist Jacob Moreno, who held his first psychodrama session in 1921. He came to believe in psychodrama because of his appreciation of group therapy and his own interest in the theatrical arts. The idea behind psychodrama is that by using dramatic techniques, a person will find the truth. That they will be able to see the way they behave with others and in situations and help people be able to deal with the emotional issues they may have in their lives. It may be used to act out past, present, or future episodes. Attacking issues in this way may give people a fresh outlook on their issues and the best way in which they can be addressed ("Psychodrama," 2016).

Psychodrama is usually performed as group therapy with one

person's experience being acted upon and the others in the group taking on other roles within that situation. However, you can perform aspects of psychodrama on your own, though it is not as simple as some of the other therapies to slot into your daily life.

There are usually three main sections to psychodrama therapy: warm-up, action, and sharing. The warm-up section is there to encourage trust and safety and ensure participants feel willing and comfortable in their surroundings and in their therapy. This may include participants introducing themselves while performing a role of some kind. In the action section, an experience in a person's life will be acted out. There are usually certain methods used to achieve this, which include:

- **Role Reversal:** A person does not play themselves but plays someone else of importance in their lives. This can bring a better understanding of why the "someone else" may behave as they do, therefore creating empathy; it may better help the person understand their relationship with the "someone else."

- **Mirroring:** The person becomes an onlooker while other people act out an experience from the person's life. This can be useful if a person is feeling quite detached from their being, is not in touch with their emotions and feelings, or if a person is feeling exceptionally negative about the experience.

- **Doubling:** Someone else takes on the person's role and expresses what they think the person's thoughts and feelings may be. This method can be used to either build an understanding of the person or to challenge, in a nice way, the manner in which the person is behaving in this scenario.

- **Soliloquy:** In a group therapy situation, this would be performed to the other members of the group or to a therapist. However, this is one you can do on your own, and if you need an audience, you can always do this with your partner, family member, or close friend—as long as whatever you are speaking about does not directly concern them. You can even use an empty chair at which you can express your feelings.

The sharing section is when the person walks through and tries to better understand what has just happened and why, how to better resolve things in the present, or how to better resolve the same types of scenarios in the future.

I think psychodrama is one of the least comfortable therapies for a person to put themselves through—particularly if you have been through traumatic events. However, for those who either really struggle to bring out their emotions or for those who, perhaps, need to reign in their emotions, it can be one of the most rewarding therapies.

A study on the effectiveness of psychodrama on middle school girls who had undergone trauma found that it reduced anxiety and depression, and the girls became less withdrawn (Carbonelli & Parteleno-Barehmi, 2016). Another study reported that psychodrama could be an effective treatment for adolescents with trauma (Mertz, 2013). Research carried out on people at an addiction center who had PTSD found that after undergoing psychodrama, there was a 25% reduction in their PTSD symptoms (Giacomucci & Marquit, 2020).

As we've seen, psychodrama is primarily a group therapy, but it is possible to conduct exercises on your own. All you need is an empty chair; the chair represents the other person in your life that this scenario is dealing with. Move the chair appropriately; place the chairs close together if you feel close to the person. If you feel distant from the person, place the chairs far apart. Then, sit down in the chair that represents you, pretend the other person is sitting in the other chair, and say everything you feel you need to say to that person. It could be there are questions you want to ask—not just express a feeling. Once you have done this, get up and go sit in the other chair and play the role of the other person, perhaps giving answers to the questions or responding to what you have said. Then, finally, go and sit back in your chair and be you again, and respond to what the other person has said. You can then carry on back and forth until you get to the resolution you need. You may want to record the conversation, as sometimes, it can be quite a shock what you may say either as yourself or the other person. This should only go on for a matter of minutes, though. This type of exercise can be so helpful if there are feelings or situations that have become unresolved. Often, it can be useful when the person you have those unresolved feelings toward is no longer with us, as you would never have the opportunity in real life to have that conversation. Whatever the situation, this exercise can be really helpful in addressing those unresolved issues and feelings, helping you feel better about yourself and other people, and making you determined to move forward in your life.

EYE MOVEMENT DESENSITIZATION AND REPROCESSING (EMDR)

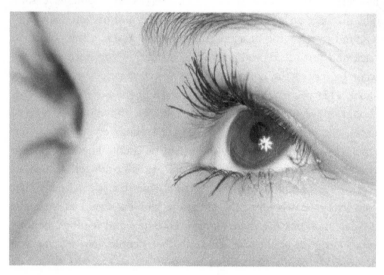

EMDR is a therapy that looks to heal people from trauma. EMDR works on the theory that just like the body would try to heal a wound, the brain, too, needs to heal from a traumatic event. When it doesn't get to heal and process properly, that is when mental health issues occur. EMDR helps reactivate that healing process.

As the name strongly hints, eye movements are used during the therapy. A person undergoing EMDR will think about certain things related to an experience while making specific movements with their eyes. Doing this helps the person begin to process these memories and feelings. Rather than feeling negatively toward these memories, they begin to feel positive at having gotten through such experiences. Eye movement works because of the similar function that occurs in your sleep with rapid eye movement (REM). Yes, that is where the band took their name from if you didn't already know that.

EMDR concentrates on the past, present, and future. It looks at the traumatic experiences of the past, the issues of the present, and the resolutions that can be achieved in the future.

There are eight phases that take place during EMDR. These are:

- **1: History Taking:** The individual works out which experiences can potentially be treated with EMDR. They may also think about what skills or changes in behavior they may need in the future to address such issues.

- **2: Identifying Tools to Cope With Emotional Distress:** A person may learn different techniques and strategies to help reduce stress between each EMDR session.

- **3, 4, 5, and 6: The EMDR Therapy:** An experience is identified and put through EMDR therapy. During this, a person will recognize an image to associate with the experience, the person's negative feelings about themselves, and any associated feelings—both physically and mentally. They will then develop positive feelings about themselves. The person will consider that positive feeling compared to the negative feeling. The person will then concentrate on the image, the negative feeling, and the bodily feelings while undergoing EMDR. This may include taps and listening to tones. The person will note how they naturally respond to these things. After each section of movements, taps, or tones, the person will try to let their mind go blank and take note of whatever first comes into their mind. The outcome of that will determine what kind of EMDR is next employed.

- **7: Close:** The person keeps a log throughout the week detailing anything relevant that occurs. It is used to reaffirm the activities the person developed to cope with things in the second phase.

- **8: Progress Report:** The final phase is reporting on the progress made.

A study of 24 trials concluded that EMDR has positive effects with regard to the treatment of emotional trauma. Seven out of the ten studies found it more effective than CBT (Shapiro, 2014). I do need to add that the study was written by Francine Shapiro, who conceived and developed EMDR, so you need to bear that in mind when considering the findings. There are further studies, though. One systematic literature review identified that EDMR improves trauma symptoms (Valiente-Gomez et al., 2017). Another analysis of all the data regarding EDMR trials concluded that EMDR therapy reduced the symptoms of PTSD significantly (Chen et al., 2014).

EMDR is another therapy where it can be best to find a therapist to work with, but it can still be worked on by yourself in the comfort of your own home. Here is an exercise to prove it:

EMDR EXERCISE #1

If you sit down somewhere comfortably, cross your hands over your chest so you are making a butterfly shape with your fingers pointing up. Then, link your two thumbs together. Use your hands to tap alternately on your chest's left and right sides. You are doing this so that your brain's left and right sides form a connection. Take note of your surroundings and anything going on. All of this should help calm you and give you a feeling of peace. It should also help you cope with and process whatever your current issue causing you stress might be.

7

SHAME TRAUMA: HEALING THE INNER CHILD AND CREATING BOUNDARIES

The trauma of shame is something that, sadly, occurs far too often and is usually linked to experiences that took place in someone's childhood. It can be hard to seek help and deal with the emotions and feelings that often manifest. But if you do, somatic healing therapy can help alleviate some of the pain.

HEALING THE INNER CHILD THROUGH SOMATIC THERAPY

Shame, like any trauma, gets "stuck" in a person. They find it hard to move on from that moment and release the shame, so it remains within, causing tension in the same way any trauma does. Shame, though, tends not to be caused by one specific incident like a car crash or a war but occurs slowly, over time, incident by incident, making the person feel like there is something wrong with them and they have no worth in the world. They start to believe that everything that goes wrong in their life is down to them. All their problems are nobody's fault but their own. Sometimes, of course, a small helping of shame can be a good thing. You did something embarrassing when you were drunk, and you wake up the next day feeling ashamed, so you call those you impacted and apologize. Shame, in that respect, helps us reassess our behavior and relationships with people, but toxic shame is not like that. It is larger in scale and a repeated incident chipping away at us until our bodies and minds can no longer deal with it. It often feels as though there is no process to reassess or take any action to move on from the shame.

For a person to deal with their shame trauma, they need to feel like they are in a comfortable, safe space. This is important for trauma generally but even more so for shame. Often, the person may have to deal with their deepest, darkest feelings, and that can only be done in a safe space where they feel comfortable enough to open up about such things.

There are a number of reasons why somatic healing therapy, in particular, is effective for shame. One is that it's very much rooted in dealing with the present, getting a person to think about the here and now, and being aware of their bodies. It's about listening to their bodies and not just their minds. With shame, it is easy for a person to become disconnected from their bodies and stop paying much attention to the details of what is happening around them. Somatic therapy is good at breaking that habit.

The other thing it's useful for, which we covered in a previous chapter, is pendulation. It's getting a person to go back and forth, from one state of being to the other, and not getting stuck in just one state. Those dealing with shame are most definitely stuck, and pendulation can help them move out of that state slowly and safely.

While there is a built-in feeling of shame within us, it is not really possible to feel shame unless someone has shamed us. It is exceptionally important for anyone going through this type of trauma to realize that the shame is being put on you. It is not your fault in any way, shape, or form. This feeling of shame is most commonly put upon us by people in power, whether that be family, friends, relationships, or work, to name a few. In fairness to those in power in our lives, they often do not realize what they are doing, but nevertheless, it is them putting the shame upon us. Equally, any neglect or an easily dismissed child can grow up with feelings of shame, which can easily be triggered later on in life.

One of the strange elements of shame is that often when people feel shamed, they then try to shame others. We may shame somebody because they have reignited the shame in us. However, the solution to losing that feeling of shame is often to go back to the original reason for it. Sadly, that can routinely be shame passed down from guardians or caregivers. They don't always think about the consequences their behavior will have and how long that impact can last for.

Many believe that the best way to finally relieve yourself of the shame is to hand back the shame to those that shamed you. They also believe this needs to be done forcefully as, more often than not, the shame was handed out forcefully (Lyon, 2017). This doesn't have to be all at once; it can be tentative at first and build up to being forceful, but it does usually need to be forceful to have the desired effect. I must be clear as well: You do not have to give it back to the person in real life (though that can be a separate option from somatic therapy) but do so in an imaginary way. This can be difficult just as an action, but many people become hesitant because they actually feel ashamed to hand back the shame—particularly if it is to a family member or someone close. However, it needs to be made clear that there is a massive difference between calling out things when they are wrong and shaming somebody. It is also important to say that the person you are giving your shame back to, in all honesty, probably did not mean what they did or did not truly understand what they were doing and what the effect of that would be. Maybe they felt ashamed and tried to pass their shame on. The shame can also pass down many generations; maybe the caregiver that shamed you had been shamed by their caregiver. The receiver of the shame gives it back to the giver of that shame and feels a release and peace within themselves because of it.

The family we grow up in and even the society we grow up in mold our impressions and early beliefs. If they are not always positive experiences, they can become limiting beliefs, as in, "I am not good enough for this," or "I do not deserve this" type of thinking. If someone tells you often enough, "You will never amount to much," well, sure enough, you start limiting your own belief in yourself. If everyone says, "Your brother is so much better than you," you may end up believing it. That can go to society as well. If certain groups of people do not receive positive messages, is it no wonder they start questioning themselves and whether they have anything to offer the world. Once you become aware of these things, it can become such a relief. That the shame and guilt you felt wasn't genuine: It has been placed on you by those around you and by society itself. Once a person realizes this, it really can be a freeing moment.

This can even extend to the culture you are brought up in. Say you are brought up in a culture where everyone must be very macho. Everyone is saying "man up" or "boys, don't cry." Suppose you grow up in a macho culture like that. In that case, it's no surprise you will probably struggle to ever show any kind of emotion or feeling to anyone else and may be somewhat aggressive in most situations you find yourself in. All of these types of things can influence our inner child and make life difficult for us when we are older. Seeing as the Taliban have just taken back over Afghanistan, perhaps you live in a culture and society where the education of women is not valued. Perhaps over time, some individuals are brainwashed into believing this absurd doctrine. Someone asks you, "Why don't you do what it is you really want to do with your own life?" You reply, "No, that is not what I'm meant to do. I am not capable of that," but you are. Society has placed a limiting belief on yourself, and you start to believe it. You end up doing things that you never really wanted to do because you believe that is right for you, and if you follow a different path, you will feel shame.

Even if we consciously reject those values and beliefs that we thought were once true and we now realize are false, there is still the issue of our subconscious mind. It is estimated that the subconscious mind is responsible for 90% of our feelings and behaviors and that a conscious decision or action is usually preceded by an unconscious one (Meyer, 2020).

The subconscious mind is extraordinary, really. If you think about when you are a baby, this is the motor that is running you. We don't really have a conscious mind until we are around five or six. It is the subconscious mind that is entirely in control of what we do up until that point. It's like a sponge soaking up everything that is going on around it and then processing it. It is inevitable that it has a heavy influence over the conscious mind.

When we are very young, our minds will normally take on any new information and take it at face value because we do not have a set of values and beliefs and lived experiences at which to judge it against. This is why those early years are so important and can have a lasting impact on us for the rest of our lives. Once we get to five or six, we now have a value and belief system to judge any new information against, and that is what our subconscious does. Hence, it is often the way we see the world at this stage in life that impacts how we see it later in life.

The inner child, then, can be seen as part of our subconscious mind. The experiences and, possibly, trauma we went through during those early years don't just get forgotten about—never to be seen again. It all gets bundled up into a small part of who we are and influences our health and happiness throughout life.

However, if that inner child is hurting or angry, and that is having a negative impact on our lives, it doesn't mean we can't do anything about our subconscious and our inner child. This is where somatic experiencing really comes into play. Previously, all this stuff was going on, and we weren't even aware. But through somatic experiences, we become aware of ourselves and our bodies. We are listening to ourselves and our bodies. Therefore, we can make a conscious effort to reprogram our subconscious with positive and loving thoughts. This can be the way we talk to ourselves, the people we surround ourselves with, and even things like social media. For all those negative thoughts and feelings you either have about yourself or hear from other people, we have to think of the positive instead. If you call yourself stupid, try to think a more positive thought. The conscious can override the subconscious if we just tell it enough times; eventually, our subconscious will start to be aligned with our conscious. Combined with all the many somatic techniques that there are, the inner child will start to feel the love, attention, and comfort it needs, and the healing process can begin.

Going through all the experiences that we do usually results in us carrying around emotional baggage. We don't mean to, but it is our way of saying, "Look at what happened to me: so many things!" It is only once we let go of our emotional baggage that we realize just how much it was weighing us down. We need to let go of that as well. Life is just too short to carry that baggage around and take it into every new situation, experience, and relationship. It is exhausting. We need to be lighter on our feet and freer in our thoughts and feelings if we are going to get anywhere near living the dream life that we want to.

We don't just need to clear out our emotional baggage, but we need to clear away those limiting beliefs. While they are still hanging around, we have no chance of healing ourselves because our minds will always be giving us reasons we can't do things. "I'm not good enough for this, so why try?" "I'm not good enough for them, so better to end it now before they realize," or "I'm just not a very sociable person, so I don't need friends." All of these kinds of thoughts and more put us off from achieving our potential as our limiting beliefs try to sabotage whatever opportunities may be out there for us. They are not the truth. To become truly self-aware, you have to realize these beliefs for what they are. Help is at hand, though. The subconscious mind producing all these thoughts of inadequacy can be reprogrammed using the emotional freedom technique (EFT) tapping. This involves tapping on various points of the body where it is believed energy fields are residing, combined with specific words or phrases to give a new message to your subconscious and reprogram it.

The conditioning and programming you go through as a child can come back and continue to haunt you through your teenage and adult years. If your role models are telling you that you are not good enough, then it wouldn't be surprising if, in your adult life, feelings of inadequacy and worthlessness start to manifest themselves. Equally, if all people around you worry about money, then in adult life, you too will probably spend your time worrying about money and chasing money. What we go through as children during those all-important stages can define us for the rest of our lives.

However, there are plenty of somatic practices that can help you to reprogram your subconscious, heal your inner child, and slowly begin to undo all that bad work that started when you were a very young child. The breathwork that has been discussed in this book can help you start to get in touch with your inner child, feel in the moment, and listen to what your inner child is saying. Things like journaling or writing a letter to your inner child can really help with dealing with this. EFT and other tapping exercises can help reprogram that subconscious and get you to say positive things about yourself and slowly remove all those negative thoughts and limiting beliefs.

One aspect of somatic therapy that has come out of looking at the inner child is the theory of "reparenting." You now have the opportunity to give yourself things you didn't get as a child that you needed by reparenting yourself—perhaps it is self-belief or compassion or any number of things. It doesn't mean your parents or caregivers were terrible at parenting, by the way: It just means they were acting out on their own beliefs and value system, and maybe they didn't give you everything you needed through no particular fault of their own.

There are forms of reparenting psychotherapy that require a therapist who will take on the role of the parent, but the essence of reparenting you can do yourself: Love yourself unconditionally. You need to be compassionate to yourself; don't judge or criticize your thoughts and feelings but legitimize them and appreciate that they are part of who you are. You give your inner child plenty of positive affirmations to remind yourself that you are loved, you are worthy, and what you think and feel is valid. If taking yourself back to your inner child and thinking about those things is too overwhelming, then you should seek out a therapist so that the exercises can be conducted in safety. But the general principles of reparenting—that you get in touch with your inner child, address the needs, and fulfill those needs—you can carry out on your own.

Learning to heal your inner child can make a world of difference for you. Having that self-compassion and the knowledge of how to take care of yourself can lead to many improved relationships—whether it be personal, family, friends, or work. You'll actually like yourself; enjoy being in your own company and the company of others, and find you enjoy life and want to live it to its fullest. You'll have confidence in yourself and your abilities, and you will have released all that pain and tension that had been holding you back for so many years. In some cases, you may have completely detached yourself from feelings and emotions, so healing the inner child will put you back in touch with yourself, and you will once again feel things like joy and love.

If healing your inner child is something you believe you need and are interested in, here is a straightforward EFT tapping exercise to set you on your way:

- **1:** First, tap the side of your hand—the side with your little finger on it rather than the thumb side—at a fairly regular pace. While tapping, say to yourself, *"I love my* *inner child. I accept my inner child. I unconditionally and without exception love myself."*

- **2:** Now, tap the top of your head, tap your forehead above your inner right eyebrow, and tap your right temple, repeating the following phrase (or a phrase you made up that fits you better) on each area: *"I love the inner child that did not get everything they needed. That child was and is incredible."*

- **3:** Tap your cheekbone, just below your eye and to the side of your nose: *"My inner child is capable of anything and has the potential to achieve anything."*

- **4:** Tap your top lip—the part in between your nose and mouth: *"My inner child does not know any limitations."* Tap your chin: *"and I love my inner child no matter what."*

- **5:** Tap below your armpit, on the side of your ribs; tap the top of your head; tap your forehead above your inner right eyebrow; and tap your right temple, repeating the following phrase on each area: *"If my inner child makes mistakes or errors, it really does not matter. I love my inner child regardless."*

- **6:** Tap your cheekbone; tap your top lip: *"I fully accept my inner child in a way that was not available at the time."*

- **7:** Tap your chin: *"I envision holding my inner child and telling them how amazing they are and that everything is going to be alright."*

- **8:** Tap the area where your heart is—toward the left of your chest: *"I will always protect my inner child and always provide protection to my inner child."*

- **9:** Tap below your armpit, on the side of your ribs: *"My inner child has my full support and acceptance."*

- **10:** Tap the top of your head; tap your forehead above your inner right eyebrow: *"I love my inner child exactly as they are."*

- **11:** Tap your right temple: *"If anyone says anything bad against my inner child, then I will stand up to them."*
- **12:** Tap your cheekbone; tap above your top lip: *"I will show my inner child that they are of value, they are worthy, and they will always be wanted and loved."*
- **13:** Tap your chin; tap your heart area: *"I really want to encourage my inner child to show just how incredible and dazzling they are."*
- **14:** Tap below your armpit, on the side of your ribs; tap the top of your head: *"By healing my inner child, I am also bringing healing to myself."*
- **15:** Tap your forehead above your inner right eyebrow: *"I no longer require the programming and conditioning that I was brought up with. What I tell myself now is the truth."*
- **16:** Tap your right temple; tap your cheekbone; tap your top lip: *"My inner child is and always will be a part of me, and when I am taking good care of myself, then I am taking good care of my inner child."*
- **17:** Tap your chin: *"When I am demonstrating love to myself, I am also loving my inner child."*
- **18:** Tap your heart area; tap below your armpit on the side of your ribs: *"When I show myself compassion, I am also being compassionate to my inner child."*
- **19:** Tap the top of your head: *"I am releasing the trauma and tension in my body and mind."*
- **20:** Tap your forehead above your inner right eyebrow: *"Release it from every bone and muscle in my body."*
- **21:** Tap your right temple: *"No more will I have to carry this emotional baggage around. It is gone forever."*
- **22:** Tap your cheekbone; tap your top lip. *"I feel so free when I release all of the pain and tension."*
- **23:** Tap your chin: *"I can't wait to see what the future holds. I am excited about the days in front of me now that I understand myself better and am in touch with myself and my inner child."*

- **24:** Tap your heart area; tap your armpit: *"I am no longer fearful, I am no longer doubtful of myself, and I look forward to seeing how the new me will take on the world."*
- **25:** Then, stop and just take a moment to relax. Take a deep breath in, and then let the breath out.

That is your tapping exercise which hopefully has been very helpful. If doing these exercises becomes too overwhelming, then seek out a professional therapist to safely help you through the process. It often helps if you can visualize your inner child when you are doing this. If you have a photo of yourself as a child, that can sometimes assist with visualization. Then you can imagine loving that child and wanting to protect that child. The next time you feel like being harsh with yourself, overly judgmental, or hyper-critical, you can look at the photo and the child's innocence. Those feelings of wanting to love and protect that child, guide them, support them, and encourage them should return. It would be advisable to repeat the exercise as often as possible. Doing it just once likely won't have the extraordinary compounding effect that daily practice will. Just find a comfortable, peaceful place for a few minutes in your day, and go through your tapping exercise. Be excited about the powerful positive results EFT tapping can provide. Remember, you can tailor the phrases to match your particular situation.

SHAME

It's scarily easy to find yourself feeling shame. You feel like you do not belong among the people you interact with. You feel like nobody understands you or could ever understand you. Shame can also come about from much more serious situations like abuse or neglect where the victim ends up feeling ashamed (when it should be the perpetrator who should be ashamed of their actions) of what has happened to them and that they let it happen. Even though, realistically, they could not have done anything to stop it. People who get ostracized at school or find themselves being bullied can often develop feelings of shame. In order to heal from shame, we need to recognize the underlying needs behind that feeling of shame.

It doesn't just happen on its own, either. Shame develops through the interconnections with others and the environment we live in. That means realizing we are not alone in the world. We are all going through a journey, working out what it means to be human. None of us really understand it or have it down perfectly. It's important to stop and appreciate that.

Shame most often occurs when our expectations of joy and happiness are not matched. For example, a child does something to a parent, and they show no interest whatsoever, or you tell a joke to your friends and nobody laughs (no wonder comedians are known to sometimes have mental health issues). Shame can surface in the forms of blushing and shyness and can include humiliation and embarrassment. Hence, such things as bullying and belittling can result in shame. As previously mentioned, shame can definitely result from something as harrowing as abuse or neglect, but it can also be from the buildup of smaller (but no less authentic) episodes.

That is not to say we should ever be without shame. Shame holds a purpose. Without it, we may never realize when we have done something wrong and would not be able to carry ourselves in society. But when shame becomes trauma, it does not serve the purpose it exists for. If it remains untreated and is left to fester in a person, then it can end up in addiction and depression, among other things. Those feeling such extreme shame usually struggle with relationships as they are expecting rejection anyway, so they try their best to get the other person out of their life first. Also, sufferers may feel very angry. So an individual trying to maintain a relationship of any kind with a sufferer whose first response is to get seriously angry, maybe even indulge in violence, is not generally a priority in life. Shame can obviously lead to feelings of insecurity and inadequacy, so this can result in things like self-harm and suicidal thoughts. Maybe someone constantly criticized ends up trying to be the perfectionist who never can attain the perfection they are after, or maybe they end up displaying symptoms of obsessive-compulsive disorder (OCD). Not only does shame cause mental issues, but it causes physical issues as well. A person with heavy shame may have bad posture, always look down and not look anyone in the eye, suffer things such as tiredness or a tightening in the chest, feel like they need to vomit, or have digestive or stomach problems.

That is, of course, where somatic therapy comes in. It can help with both the mental and the physical symptoms of shame. By becoming aware of what your body is telling you, you are likely to realize that the tension in your body relates to the shame you are feeling in your everyday life. As you think about and deal with those episodes of your life that may have contributed to this shame, release them, and let go, these episodes become signals of strength for you rather than something making you weak and fearful.

Shame nearly always relates back to what occurred in your childhood. Those insecurities, doubts, fears, and low self-esteem you feel now are likely rooted in your childhood. If you are constantly scolded for the slightest misjudgment, then it is hardly surprising if you grow up thinking everything you do is wrong or that there is something wrong with you. If you get bullied, you can develop feelings of "Why me? There must be something wrong with me." Obviously, truly traumatic experiences like abuse and neglect can bring these feelings out in a much more extreme way.

If we know that our adult feelings of shame are deeply rooted in our childhood, then we know that healing the inner child can, in turn, heal our shame. Some of the best techniques and therapies to help with this include CBT, where we learn to try to control and change our thought behaviors and patterns. Therefore, instead of thinking of insults to ourselves, we can learn to think positive thoughts and reaffirm the reality that we are good and capable of good things.

Prolonged exposure (PE) can be a good form of therapy to address this issue. Slowly, a person pays attention to things that stimulate them and makes them deal with the issue. Maybe you start with a photo of yourself as a child, then discuss your shame as a child. Then you imagine yourself somewhere that reminds you of that shame. Slowly but surely, it will remove the power the shame has over you.

Stress inoculation training can be a good therapy to employ. Rather than stress itself, it uses the same training to contain and control your shame. It can include breathing and muscle relaxation techniques, role-play, and taking note of negative thoughts and amending them. There is also such a thing as compassionate mind training (CMF), which can help a person who speaks negatively about themselves change their behavior and be compassionate and kind toward themselves and their inner child.

EMDR is another good one to follow. Thinking about your shame and all that hurt your inner child has experienced while undergoing the eye movement actions may well help to alleviate your shame and start to heal your inner child.

However, one of the most powerful techniques for healing shame and your inner child is EFT tapping. It is one of the best techniques because you don't necessarily have to relive those memories when you were shamed over and over. You just need to remember them enough to release them. EFT is, in its essence, a healing process and not a memory jukebox. Combining the positive affirmations with the tapping of the energy points on your body can be exceptionally powerful and provide a true sense of relief and release from your shame, making you realize your inner child needs love. As your inner child is part of you, it is you who can best provide that love and support.

Here's a specific EFT tapping exercise to help you learn to heal not only your shame but also your inner child. You don't have to repeat the affirmation if it does not relate to you. We all went through different experiences, so if the affirmations aren't right for you, just replace them with what you think is more appropriate to the experience you went through and the shame you feel.

- **1:** Start by tapping the side of your hand and saying, *"I may not have received the love and belief that I needed as a child, but I still love and accept myself. Although I may feel that I am not worthy and insult myself and doubt myself, I still wholeheartedly love and accept myself."*
- **2:** Tap the top of your head, your forehead above your inner right eyebrow, the side of your temple, your cheekbone, your top lip under your nose, your chin, your heart area, and under your armpit at the side of your ribs. Do this cycle approximately eight times while saying the following:

  I may not have felt supported when I was a child or felt like there was someone there for me all the time. I may not have felt there was anybody to protect me, and I may have suffered terrible consequences as a result. I always thought there was either something wrong with me or that everything I did was wrong. I always felt I deserved the bad things that happened to me. I just didn't know any better back then.

  I say negative things about myself. I sometimes get so embarrassed by myself that I detest myself. Sometimes, I see myself in the mirror, and I really do not like what I see. When I think about my life, I feel like I have achieved nothing, and everything I have done amounts to nothing. I give myself unrealistic expectations and targets to meet. It makes me feel like I don't see the point of anything. These are all things that I have built into my being since I was a young child. Although this is what I learned as a child, I have now learned that my belief that I am not worthy is utterly false.

As a child, I did not know any better, though, so I believed it to be true for many years; that lie still influences my life today. When these thoughts enter my head, it makes me feel very low and unhappy. I must have the strength and courage to change these thoughts as I know. Now that I am an adult, I know these thoughts are not the truth. My mind may now realize this, and the tapping I am now doing will tell it to my heart and the rest of my body. I know all these thoughts I had about myself are wrong and untrue, but they made me feel like there was something wrong with me and like no one could possibly love me.

I could never be good enough for someone else. All untrue. I no longer have to carry around the emotional baggage that my caregivers handed to me. The shame that my caregivers possessed and passed to me goes no further. It stops here. They can keep the shame. I reject it. It is acceptable that I am not perfect in every way, and I have flaws. This is what being human is. I love myself, and I accept myself—flaws and all. The shame I once felt no longer has any hold over me. When I release the shame, I feel free, and I feel relieved. I look forward to the new relationship I have with myself.

- **3:** Take a deep breath in, breathe out, and relax.

SETTING HEALTHY BOUNDARIES WITH SOMATIC SKILLS

Setting boundaries can be essential in helping yourself heal and recover from trauma. They are the mechanisms that separate you from other people. It is what helps define you as you—where you begin and where you end. Boundaries are meant to be flexible, though. When you feel safe, you are more likely to extend those boundaries, and when you don't feel safe, you will restrict and pull those boundaries in. You can see how this is important. If your boundaries are too free, you end up giving yourself to others, and it can be easy to lose yourself. On the contrary, if your boundaries are too restricted, then you can become isolated from the rest of the world and become lonely.

Like most things, our boundaries were learned from how our caregivers responded to us when we were children. They should engage with us when we need engagement and leave us alone when we need space. It is not always a problem if caregivers don't engage: This can help the child strengthen their resolve and ability to cope. However, there are three main areas where if caregivers overstep the mark, it can cause issues:

- **1: Invasion:** This is where the caregiver, rather than letting a child have their "alone" time, will do the opposite. Maybe because they need their comfort, not for any malicious reasons, but this can lead to a child growing up and installing very closed-off boundaries, withdrawing, and therefore, potentially becoming isolated.

- **2: Abandonment:** This is the opposite of invasion. Caregivers do not respond to a child's needs or wish for engagement. In adulthood, this can result in boundaries that are too free. A person will end up trying to please everyone, maybe always trying to do things to gain attention, and they can lose themselves within that.

- **3: Both Invasion and Abandonment:** In this scenario, the caregiver inconsistently alternates between the two. This can really cause issues because sometimes a person may end up trying to overplease people, and sometimes, they will end up pushing everybody away. It is hard enough maintaining any kind of relationship with an individual who consistently does one of these things. But, if they are doing both, sometimes randomly, it can only make life a headache both for them and those around them.

I don't really like to label people. I've always thought there is probably some truth in Becker's labeling theory, but for the sake of being clear, I am going to refer to "toxic" people—though I am sure they are good people at heart, and they just haven't had their own boundaries set for them. We all know people like this: People who have negative thoughts and feelings are the ones who always seem to find a way to bring us down or let us down. Setting boundaries is one way of not having such people in your life if you don't want them. If you have set healthy boundaries, these types of people should be nowhere near you. Equally, the kinds of conflict or awkward situations you can find yourself in can be avoided with boundary setting. If those boundaries are there, then you and everyone else know where you stand, and conflict should not be a daily occurrence.

Having somatic skills can be extraordinarily helpful in setting and maintaining boundaries. For a start, you will start to develop your body awareness. You will start to discover that "felt sense." That will help enormously in telling you whether things feel right or not and whether you need to strengthen your boundaries. You will also have that self-awareness about your own thought processes. Whereas before, you may have automatically done or said something which would have allowed someone to take advantage of you or cause you to withdraw when someone was only trying to help you out, now, you will be aware of what you are doing and how you are behaving. This may stop you from making those same errors when it comes to your boundaries.

One of the most important skills to learn for setting your boundaries is learning the ability to say "no"—not just in a half-hearted way but in a way where the other person knows you are not going to budge from that. Don't just automatically say "yes." Always think through your response, and remember to listen to that "felt sense" of yours as well. You can start off with small things like saying "no" to coming out on Friday night because you are worn out and you really just need a night in. Or saying "no" to loaning the person money when they never pay you back. That's not a loan: You are just giving them money. Next time, don't do it. Of course, people are disappointed when you say no—that is inevitable, but that doesn't mean you have to give in. You will disappoint people, but that will make them respect you more, and the next time you say "yes," they will know you really mean it, and they will stop asking you unnecessarily in the future.

This brings us to what you do need to say a definite "yes" to, and that is your commitment to healing and looking after yourself. If you are putting your needs first, respecting yourself, and loving yourself, then saying "no" to others becomes easier. Say "no" to others but "yes" to yourself.

Here's an exercise to help with your boundary setting, which will help you in saying "yes" and "no" and ensuring your body is saying the same thing.

BOUNDARY EXERCISE #1

First, see what happens to your body when you say "yes" out loud. Repeat it several times and see what you notice. Now, try saying "yes" with your body instead. What changes? Maybe it is your breathing or your posture. Is your movement free? Do you feel tense? Think about and note down the situations in which you would like to be able to say "yes." For example, do you want to do a boundary-setting exercise? "Yes!"

Next, do the same but for saying "no." Take note of how your body responds to you saying "no" out loud several times. Then, try saying "no" just with your body and see what changes there are in your body. Think about the situations in which you would like to be able to say "no." For example, "Are you coming out again tonight?"

Take one of the situations where you said you would like to say "yes," take on the body posture of saying "yes," and note down what occurs when you imagine that scenario. Then, do the same with a situation you want to say "no" to.

At the end of that, you should be aware of how to ensure your body and voice are saying the same thing and being really clear about what you are communicating.

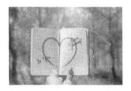

8

ANXIETY, SELF-LOVE, SELF-COMPASSION, AND CRUSHING DEPRESSION

E verything that is mentioned in this title, somatic therapy can address and resolve. If you find you have anxiety, then this is something that somatic therapy can treat. If you have depression, then this is something that somatic therapy can crush into the dust. If you are in desperate need of learning how to show love and compassion to yourself, somatic therapy can show you how and help you achieve that. Do you want to be able to forgive yourself for doing things that you perceive to have been wrong? Somatic therapy can help you find that release of negativity from your soul. Somatic therapy is like finding a water fountain in the middle of a desert. You have a thirst for healing yourself, and somatic therapy is going to quench that thirst for you.

It's hard to move on, though, if you don't give yourself a break. You need to be able to forgive yourself. No one is perfect, and that includes you. You made some mistakes and errors in life, but we all have. That's all part and parcel of the human experience. If you don't find room in your heart to forgive yourself, you will never get past the first obstacle. You will always feel resentment. You will always be prone to anger and lashing out at your nearest and dearest. You will never achieve what you want to in life or reach your maximum potential. You need to clear your heart and forgive yourself; then, you can start to look at all the exciting opportunities there are for you in life.

You also need to practice detachment from outcomes. Once you do that, it will help you clear your heart, forgive yourself, and stand a chance to reach your maximum potential. Best of all, you might actually enjoy life rather than worrying about it all the time! I found when I practiced detachment, it really did free me up from so much stress and worry that I was previously focused on. Realize that you cannot control everybody else. People will let you down, and people will do things you don't agree with. That, I'm afraid, is life. You can't fix those people. The only person you can "fix" is yourself. You don't need fixing because there isn't really anything wrong with you; you need healing. The only person's actions that you are ever in control of are your own.

Find your own version of happiness. Don't take any notice of other people telling you whether you should be happy or not or trying to define your achievements or lack of them. It's down to you to decide what true happiness looks like—not anybody else. However, you also need to detach from the idea that everything has to work out a certain way because it doesn't. Look how often you plan an event only for something completely out of our control to change that. The pandemic is a prime example of that. Out go all our plans due to something out of our control. Accept it: Things do not need to be a certain way or the perfect way. Once you can accept that, you will find you truly feel free to enjoy and appreciate life. Also, you probably won't be as hard on yourself in the future as well. You won't just enjoy and appreciate life, but you will enjoy and appreciate being you.

Let's give ourselves some self-love right now with a quick EFT tapping exercise:

- **1:** Start off by tapping the side of your hand as you say: "I accept myself for who I am. I love myself for who I am. I respect myself, and I expect others to respect me as well. I love myself fully. I do have value. I do have worth. I am good enough. I do deserve to have love and to be loved. I honestly do love myself, and I promise to love and respect myself. I accept myself as the person that I am."

- **2:** Tap your inner forehead above your right eyebrow; tap the side of your temple; tap your cheekbone: "I completely love myself. I respect myself, and I believe I am of great value."

- **3:** Tap your top lip; tap your chin; tap under your armpit on the side of your ribs: "Loving myself is a magnificent thing to do. Thinking that I could not love myself is no longer an option."

- **4:** Tap the top of your head, your forehead, your temple, your cheekbone, your top lip, your chin, your heart area, and under your armpit: "Some of my behavior was probably because of this incorrect belief that I could not love myself. But now, my mind and heart are open to the potential of self-love. Maybe I was scared to love myself previously, but I reject that notion now. I am not afraid. I am ready to love myself."

- **5:** Tap the top of your head; tap your forehead; tap your temple; tap your cheekbone: "I find that, actually, the more I love myself, that I love myself even more."

- **6:** Tap your top lip; tap your chin: "By loving myself, I find it makes it easier to love others."

- **7:** Tap your heart area; tap under your armpit: "This makes me happy. That's why I love loving myself."

- **8:** Tap the top of your head; tap your forehead; tap your temple. "I reject all the thoughts I previously had that made me believe I could not love myself."

- **9:** Tap your upper lip; tap your chin; tap your heart area;

tap your head: "I clean my heart and forgive myself in order to be able to love myself."

- **10:** Tap under your armpit: "I love and value myself. I deserve respect. I will love myself because I deserve love."
- **11:** Take a deep breath in, breathe out, and relax.

To go alongside self-love, you need self-compassion, so here is an EFT tapping exercise for self-compassion. I suggest you complete the tapping cycle approximately three times while saying the words below:

> I will be compassionate toward myself. I love and accept myself for who I am. I love myself; therefore, I will be compassionate toward myself. Since I am compassionate toward myself, I will look after myself and care for myself. I love myself wholeheartedly. I clear my heart—ready to take on the compassion I now have for myself. All the thoughts and reasons I held before that made me not be compassionate toward myself I now reject. I release those negative thoughts and feelings from my mind and from my body. It's great for me to show compassion toward myself. It will make me healthier both in mind and body, and it will make me a better person. If I am compassionate toward myself, then I am more likely to show genuine compassion for others as well. I refute talking negatively about myself or putting myself down. I realize now that that was not a healthy way to be. The next time I make an error of judgment or I make a mistake, I will show myself compassion. I deserve to be compassionate toward myself, and I will be compassionate toward myself.

Take a deep breath in, breathe out, and relax.

We've given ourselves some self-love and self-compassion, and now it's time for some self-forgiveness. If we don't practice this, we will always be angry at ourselves and the world. Let's begin the healing and forgive ourselves. Repeat the tapping cycle approximately three times for this while saying:

> *I want to forgive myself thoroughly. I feel ashamed about things I have said or done in the past. I want to release the guilt and tension I have and feel free. It is alright for me to forgive myself. In order to let go and be free, I need to forgive myself. I wholeheartedly love and accept myself, and I forgive myself. If I love myself, then it follows that I can forgive myself. If I want to look after myself, then it follows that I forgive myself. I deserve forgiveness even if I fight against that belief sometimes. I love myself unconditionally; therefore, I forgive myself. Whatever I have done in the past, I accept the blame. I learned from those mistakes I made in the past. Now, I forgive myself, and I move on from it. I'm looking forward to beginning afresh now that I have forgiven myself—to live a happier and healthier life and to be able to forgive myself and forgive others with ease. I accept myself as I am, and I forgive myself. I fully forgive myself. I am a good person. I forgive myself, and I am at peace with myself.*

Take a deep breath in, breathe out, and relax.

I know that the words "self-love" can either bring out images of people with round, purple sunglasses and flowers in their hair or make you think it is a euphemism of some kind. Yet there's a reason the phrase, "You can't love somebody else until you love yourself," exists. The fact is that until you love yourself, it makes dealing with the rest of the world a lot harder. If you hate yourself, it is almost inevitable that you will feel angry with yourself and everyone else because there has to be some kind of outlet to get that anger out. If you don't love yourself, then you don't respect yourself, so you will always put someone else's needs and wants before your own. If this is in work, it will probably lead you to face complete burnout. If it's relationships, your personality and individualism will probably become completely subsumed by your partner. If you love yourself, then when those bad things in life happen (which they will—there's no escaping some of them, such as the death of a loved one), then you are so much better equipped to deal with situations in a healthy way and not resort to unhealthy ways to get through them. Once you develop self-love, then everything else comes from it: respect, value, confidence, and belief; those other things we talked about, like compassion and forgiveness for yourself, become so much easier.

Of course, it's not easy to get to that point. There are so many blocks and obstacles that we put in the way of ourselves getting to that point. It's all the negative talk and limiting beliefs that we place before ourselves, believing we are not good enough, not worthy of love, and will never amount to anything. We need to clear our hearts and minds of those thoughts and feelings to progress to self-love.

Once we love ourselves, then the opportunity to forgive ourselves becomes possible. Although, we need to take responsibility, own up to, and apologize for genuinely bad things we've done and said. However, if you're looking in this book, then the likelihood is you are blaming yourself when it really wasn't your fault. As the saying goes, "It takes two to tango." Whatever the situation is— you think you hurt someone or upset someone—it took two to make that happen. You can't just do it all by yourself, so it can't all possibly be your fault. Unless you were in a tango dance, and then you stepped on your partner's foot, then that was your fault. No, hang on: "It takes two to tango."

You are not alone either; we all have made terrible errors and judgments in our lives. We make thousands of decisions every day, so it is inevitable that some of them don't go as well as we would hope. That's life. If you can make that step to forgiving yourself, it truly is transformational. Once you realize not everything is your fault, not everything is down to you, and not everything is based on what you do, that can really change things for you. Until you do that, sadly, you are probably going to stop yourself from living the best possible life you can. There is always going to be an element of self-sabotage, but once you forgive yourself and let go of all that self-doubt and self-blame, then anything becomes possible.

Let's do an EFT tapping exercise to clear the blame. You know the score by now. Start with some tapping on the side of your hand. Then move through the cycle from the top of your head to the side of your ribs. Tap for as long as feels right, or as long as you need to. Say the following:

> *I'm embarrassed about what I have done and said. It was so silly of me to do. I regret my actions very much and feel very guilty about it. I would like to be able to forgive myself for it, but I still feel it is all my own fault. Thus far, I have not been able to let go of the guilt and forgive myself. Today that changes. With this tapping, I am starting my journey of releasing the guilt and shame from my mind and body. Today, I forgive myself, and I no longer hold on to the guilt. I love and accept myself, so I know I can make that step to forgiving myself. Not everything is my fault; not everything happens because of me and the way I am. I know that now. I didn't before. Hence, I was unable to forgive myself. I will now forgive myself. If I could turn back time, I would have done things differently, but I know I am human. Whatever was causing me to behave the way I did took place, but it is human to err. For that, I can forgive myself. All this guilt, shame, and regret that I have been holding in all these years, I now give it permission to clear. I am*

releasing it all from my body and my mind. Slowly and safely, I release it all. I am ready to forgive myself. I let go of all my guilt. I clear my guilt from my head and heart.

Take a deep breath in, breathe out, and relax.

Even with all these promises of forgiveness and self-love to ourselves, it can be challenging to move past a certain point. That is because we sometimes have internal conflict going on within us. We want to forgive ourselves, but something stops us and says, "No, you don't deserve forgiveness." Generally, internal conflict can sometimes just mean things don't feel right within us. We are not at peace with ourselves or with someone else. If that internal conflict is not resolved, it can turn into much more serious afflictions such as despair and depression. You need to be able to clear that inner conflict within yourself in order to be able to progress.

Everything around this chapter—and the entire book—is about exploring yourself and finding out about yourself. It's about how you've been programmed over the years and how you have had limiting beliefs put on you. It's about how you can learn to love yourself, accept yourself, and forgive yourself. Through this self-discovery, it will become clear why you have behaved the way you have and why you have had these feelings and emotions over the years. Maybe you will even discover new emotions and feelings you didn't even know were in you. Up until now, you have, at best, been treading water, barely keeping your head above the water. You have not had that opportunity to really grab life's opportunities and think about what it is you are really meant to be doing. There is a word in Sanskrit—*dharma*—which takes on the kind of meaning of what your soul's purpose is. Well, in your journey of self-discovery, this is really the chance to find what the purpose of your soul and your life is. This is the chance to give your soul all the nourishment and goodness it could possibly need as you explore yourself and love yourself more. Now is the chance to find out what it really is that you want to do and what it is that will make your soul sing. Grab life's microphone and belt out the number your soul is longing you to. This can all be achieved with the help of somatic therapy. It can heal you, it can help you discover yourself, and it can help you move away from anxiety and depression to a true place of happiness and peace. Somatic therapy can help you achieve all of that and more.

DEPRESSION AND SOMATIC THERAPY

Depression can last for days, months, and even years. It is a challenging thing to cope with and struggle through when it's happening. It can be brought on by anything. Maybe something in your life dramatically changes, or you go through a traumatic event. Sometimes, it comes on when there doesn't appear to be a reason—your body is probably just catching up years after the event, or something small is the thing that has tipped your body over the edge. Depression is what occurs when our body goes into permanent "freeze" mode or even to its "shutdown" mode. Women tend to experience depression twice as much as men ("Depressive Disorders," n.d.). This is perhaps not that surprising considering everything their bodies and internal dynamics have to go through compared to men—combined with the pressure women often put on themselves to "have it all": a pressure that is thoroughly absent from most men's lives.

I remember the one time in my life when I really struggled with depression. It was my late teenage years to my early 20s. I can remember it very well because, although I have not had any episodes like it for many years, I am always on the lookout for the same feelings coming back. It used to be a massive effort just to get out of bed. If I got out of bed before noon, it was a miracle. Once I was up, I could not be bothered to shower, brush my teeth, or get dressed. I always wanted to be alone, as being in the company of other people became excruciating. You don't think anyone would want to be around you, so it becomes a self-fulfilling prophecy as you isolate yourself from anyone who would want to help and support you. Though I could never have carried out a suicide attempt, I just didn't have that kind of action in me; it didn't stop me from having the kind of thoughts where you don't think anyone would miss you if you weren't there, and the world would probably be a better place if you weren't there. Possibly, you'd be happier if you weren't there anymore because life is just too painful and too much effort for you. In my case, I don't think there was one event that triggered it off; I think it was many things over a long period of time that brought me to that point, and I think it was because it was a part of my life where everything was changing as well. I was questioning who I was a lot of the time. Putting it into words doesn't even begin to describe how dark and lonely depression is, but I don't feel like that now—that's the positive. If you can address it, depression does not have to last forever. There's a reason our bodies and minds go into depression, so that means there's a way out. That way can be via somatic therapy.

We already know from the previous chapters that there are many somatic therapy techniques you can try if you feel depressed. You can use CBT to challenge your thinking patterns. You can inquire into all those thoughts you are constantly having that describe the worst possible outcome or state. Let's think about how realistic that thought actually is and see if we can change the thinking pattern. Vagal nerve stimulation can be a good one as well. There are more extreme versions of that where electrodes are used to stimulate the nerve rather than just your fingers, but just doing some simple vagal nerve stimulation will get your social engagement system going. Then, you can get into a more playful mood where maybe you can play around with the expressions your face makes, the tone of voice you have, and try to get that black cloud hovering over you to move on, allowing the sunshine to burst through.

You can follow some straightforward techniques that really help with depression specifically. One is to put yourself in postures or positions where you lengthen the spine. The next chapter mentions somatic yoga practices, which include postures that are helpful to this. When we become depressed, our body tends to hunch over, and our chest caves in a bit, so doing things to lengthen your spine helps to improve your mindset and outlook. It's not a permanent cure, but it can be beneficial among all your other somatic work.

Movement is also a great thing to help you if you feel depressed. Just getting out of your chair and standing up can make a small difference. Still, if you do some basic exercise, some small yoga movements, some Qigong, or just some muscle tense and release exercises—both of which are covered in Chapter 9—it can really help lift your spirits and get you feeling a bit better about yourself.

Sensorimotor psychotherapy, which I walked you through in Chapter 6, can be a handy tool in any fight against depression. Take the time to feel your body and ask those questions to yourself about how you feel about things. Just taking the time to know your body and the world around you can perk up your nervous system and help it output some positive energy.

ANXIETY, TRIGGERS, STRESS REDUCTION, AND SOMATIC THERAPY

Anxiety is a form of extreme worrying where you feel exceptionally stressed, your breathing may become shallow, you may feel as though you will have a panic attack, you feel sick in your stomach, or your skin is itchy. Different people have different physical reactions to anxiety, but the mental anguish is similar: You are scared or worried about something or some situation. Triggers are what your memory associated with the danger—be it a person, event, or object. For example, I had a friend who used to be a landlord, and one tenant caused her a major headache. Once that tenant left, my friend became very fearful of anything to do with the apartment. She started imagining all kinds of problems with the apartment that didn't actually exist, but it wasn't the apartment that was the actual danger—it was the behavior of unpredictable people that had been the real danger. The apartment in itself was perfectly fine.

I know someone who was having chemotherapy. They celebrated their completed first round of healing by eating fish and chips—not realizing that the chemo was likely to make them sick later. Sure enough, they "were ill" after the fish and chips. Thereafter, they could not face fish and chips for a very long time—not just because it had made them sick but because it ultimately reminded them of chemo and, therefore, of cancer. These triggers can work for very ordinary objects and things, but because they relate to the danger the person encountered, the brain gets scared and links the two together, jumping to the wrong conclusion.

I should be clear: triggers are not a bad thing. Their job is important by making us aware of impending danger. An issue only starts to arise when your brain and body go into overdrive, and you start to get triggered to danger when, in fact, everything is perfectly safe. This can become a spiraling issue, where, in the example of my friend's apartment, they become fearful of it, so the best way to escape that fear is not to go near it or not talk to anybody about it. However, then your mind starts making the association that what saved you from your (imagined) danger about the apartment is not going near it. Then, you can become anxious just generally about apartments. Any apartment now is a trigger for the danger. Now, you're afraid to go out because you might see an apartment, and you try not to talk to anyone because they might mention that they live in an apartment. Although this may sound a little silly, this kind of thought cycle is not uncommon. When the triggers reach this level of sensitivity, they become the danger. You can get caught in a spiral of anxiety that only ever travels down.

Here are some straightforward and easy-to-follow somatic therapy exercises that you can use to heal your anxiety and dampen those triggers:

- **1:** You are going to get yourself into a good "grounded" position. Make sure you are sitting comfortably in a chair or on a sofa with your feet placed firmly on the floor in front of you. Try to get your shoulders, neck, and arms to relax. Place your hands and arms on your thighs so that you are in a good position to breathe. Breathe as you would normally and try to concentrate on where you are feeling the anxiety physically. Identify those areas. Is it your stomach? Is it that your chest feels tight? Is it your hands that feel sweaty? Is it that your skin feels itchy? Is it that your heart is pounding? Wherever it is that you are feeling the anxiety, concentrate on that area and imagine your breath coming from that area. You can touch the area so that your mind and body make the connection of where the anxiety is and that you want to heal it. You should be in that situation of breathing, concentrating, and healing for approximately 30 seconds to see what happens, and then you should experience that for a full minute. Hopefully, the area shoud feel less tense, and your anxiety will begin to reduce.

- **2:** Every so often, just sit down and touch base with yourself. How are you breathing? Are you breathing with your chest? Then make sure you focus, and breathe with your stomach instead. Taking away that shallow form of breathing should start to impact your feelings of anxiety and start to lessen them.

- **3:** When you are feeling tense, scrunch up that part of your body, make it as tense as possible, and then slowly let it out gently. As strange as it may seem, making the area where you are feeling the anxiety as tense as possible and then letting it go can actually reduce the anxiety. This is because your body and mind recognize an issue and address it. Once you have done this, your body may feel more relaxed. Without this method and by just trying to relax alone, your body feels like maybe you are trying to ignore it. By recognizing anxiety and scrunching up as tight as possible in the relevant area and then letting go, your body notes you have recognized it is having difficulties in that area. Now, you have recognized that it is happy to forget it and move on.

SOMATIC ANGER RELEASE

Anger is sometimes reacted to as a maligned emotion. We view it with suspicion and fear. If someone is angry, we sometimes see that as a weakness; for example, we may hear, "Oooh, what's wrong with them? Touched a nerve, did I?" and other such comments. Of course, like all emotions, anger does serve a purpose. If we are angry, it is because something is wrong. When someone is always angry, there is something wrong that's much deeper. It's not just an issue at work or irritation because your partner didn't do what you asked them to do. It can also lead a person into trouble. Constant anger could lead to violence and threats or saying unkind things to people that aren't meant to be. For some people, it can result in silent treatment or a never-ending sulk. When it comes down to it, whatever the outcome, it is just not pleasant feeling like that— being always at odds with everyone and everything. It is exhausting on top of everything else, and a person will probably not be left with many friends or family that can tolerate that permanent anger. However, I want you to remember something: It is okay to be angry, and it is not something to be ashamed of. It is a normal human emotion that we all go through. It can be dangerous to suppress emotions and can lead to health issues, so being angry is fine, within reason. We just need to be careful when the only emotion we ever seem to feel is anger.

Somatic therapy and experiencing can be such a great help to those who need to understand, release, and let go of anger in a healthy way. It will help release all those emotions buried deep inside that a person has been unwilling to recognize and accept.

Using somatic techniques over a long period of time can assist greatly in managing and regulating anger, which in turn can have the health benefits of reducing digestion issues, more relaxed muscles, better concentration, and a better night's sleep (Friedman, 2019).

As anger is such a powerful emotion, it is essential to deal with it in a safe and healthy way. Engaging in cathartic methods where someone is encouraged to let it all out with screaming or more physical releases is one way but may not be healthy. However, by using somatic experiencing and other such practices over time where you learn how to listen to your body, you can start to understand your anger. You can let it out little by little in a controlled and healthy way and in a safe space. Just letting it all out in one go in an uncontrolled manner may not have such a safe effect on you—particularly if you have PTSD or other trauma symptoms. It can actually be quite harmful to you, and any anger is only going to be released temporarily—it is not going to have the long-lasting effect you require.

Let's get into a somatic anger release exercise to see how easy it is to do; once again, it is safe to do in your own home, and you can go into a room by yourself and practice when the emotion becomes apparent.

First, as always with somatic practices, get to know your body. Take some time to feel where in your body the anger is. Take some deep breaths in and out and feel where that anger is. Now, wherever you are feeling that anger, shake your body. You can use your hands to apply some light pressure if you want to. Shake your body and imagine yourself shaking that anger out so that it is gone and you are free and ready to move on. This is a really simple, straightforward exercise for you to manage when feeling angry or frustrated.

Another option is to find something that you can squeeze very hard: a towel, some clothes, or you can even squeeze the forearm of a partner or friend. Just be careful: It is the forearm and not the wrist or elbow joint. Make sure it's something that gives you a burst of letting the anger out, so you can carry on with your day.

Combining these exercises with your general somatic experiencing will allow you to get to know your body, understand where and why the anger lives, and allow you to slowly but surely release and let it go so that you can resume and get on with your life healthily and safely.

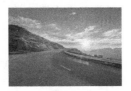

9

DISCOVER NEW ROADS TO RECOVERY (FURTHER TECHNIQUES TO HEAL TRAUMA)

While not part of somatic experiencing, there are many further techniques that are somatic in nature, and you can incorporate them into your healing and therapy routines. They all help with the brain's flexibility and spark its ability to adapt and change for the better.

QIGONG AND SHAKING PRACTICES

The translation of "Qigong" is "energy work." That's because, in its essence, what you do when you practice Qigong is to try to channel energy through your palms. Usually, this is done while standing up. This is usually combined with certain breathwork as well. The key to it all is the coordination of the eyes with the movements you make, combined with your breathing and the concentration of your mind. A review of the many studies on Qigong and Tai Chi (another practice) concluded that they had many health and psychological benefits (Jahnke et al., 2010). If you think back to what Peter Levine said about animals shaking off their trauma, it makes sense that engaging in energy practices, including shaking, can be good for our physical and mental health.

The good thing about Qigong, like so many somatic practices, is you can do it anywhere; as long as you can find a quiet and peaceful place, you can easily practice it.

To give you a flavor, here is an easy shaking practice for you to follow:

- Begin by standing up with a good, upright posture. Close your eyes and feel yourself breathing; feel yourself and your body in the present moment. Then, when you feel ready to do so, open your eyes, but be careful not to lose that feeling of being in the present; wake up the energy within your body. Start by shaking your right arm, but be sure to keep it in a relaxed state: Don't tense it up when shaking. Then, shake your right leg. You will need to lift your leg up slightly off the ground in order to do so. When you feel it is ready to move on, put your right leg down and shake your left arm. Then, when it feels right to do so, move onto your left leg.

- Once you feel it is okay to move down, put down your left leg and shake your whole body: arms, legs, body, head—everything. Again, be mindful to keep your body loose and relaxed—don't tense it all up. You can close your eyes if you want to. Unlike when you were shaking your leg, you should keep your feet on the floor. However, you can lift your heels up and down but don't actually lift your leg off from the floor. Try shaking yourself even harder, give yourself up to the act of shaking, and see if you can really release that energy from inside of you. You can lift your arms up if that is what your energy is directing you to do. Your mouth should be completely relaxed, so if this guides you to making noises, that is fine. You are letting energy out, so making some noise is fine if that is what you are directed to do. Very slowly, start to shake a little less hard—do this slowly until you are back into a static standing posture.

SOMATIC YOGA

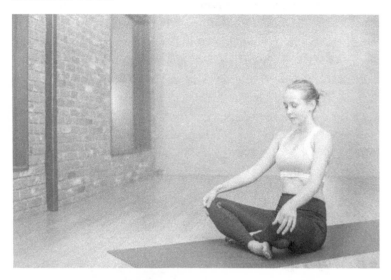

Somatic yoga is, as the name suggests, a mixture of yoga with the mind-body principles of somatics. It uses the somatic awareness of the body to help you rewire your brain and give your muscles a workout to release that tension and stress that may have built up due to trauma. You aren't just following what a yoga teacher is telling you and copying the movement. You are actually doing that movement and thinking about how your body feels and what your body is telling you.

One aspect of the somatic yoga practice is ensuring there is an element of grounding included. As you may well remember from previous chapters, grounding gives us that feeling of safety and calmness, which is so important if we are to listen to our bodies. For many of the previous practices, grounding meant sitting down with your feet firmly planted on the floor. For yoga, that is slightly different, as you can imagine. Grounding in this context consists of sitting on the floor, cross-legged, with your arms outstretched resting on your legs. Then you lift your hands up in the air, make the peace sign with both hands, and then place your hands (still in the peace sign mode) on the floor, letting your shoulders relax. You may feel the need to close your eyes. In this situation, the floor is the earth, so this grounding is us making our connection with the earth. As with all grounding, this is where you start to feel your body in the present and in the here and now. Then, you can take a deep breath in and let the breath out; then, you will be ready to begin the rest of your yoga practice.

The various poses you can do in yoga have specific reasons and benefits. I'm just going to walk through a few of them here, so you know their benefits:

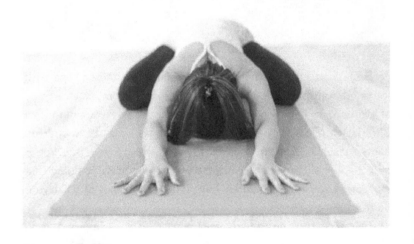

- **Child's Pose:** This pose is meant to calm you down and can be known to reduce stress and increase energy. To carry it out, you need to get into a kneeling position. Your big toes should be touching, and your knees need to be apart. Take a deep breath in and try to lengthen your spine. Breathe out and bend forward—moving your head toward the floor. If you want to, you can use your hands to rest your head on. Open the backs of your shoulders up and allow your stomach and your chest to expand. You may want to move your knees further apart. Let your arms relax and place them by your feet, with the palms facing up. Breathe and relax. You should feel the position become more pronounced when breathing. As it is a pose for relaxation, take a few minutes to stay in that position and relax. When you are ready to come out of the pose, move your hands up to your knees, breathe in, and move your hands around to use them to push into the floor and lift yourself up. Move your chest and shoulders up slowly so you are back into a kneeling position, sitting upright.

- **Standing Cat-Cow Pose:** These are actually two different poses that have been combined to make an even more effective pose. It can help with the flexibility of your spine and, therefore, your posture. However, best of all, for our purposes, it helps calm a person and can reduce stress. To do this, you need to start off on your hands and knees, with your head in the center of your body looking down. First, do the Cow Pose, so breathe in and move your stomach toward the floor while raising up your chin and chest and averting your gaze up. Try to move your shoulders outward and away from your ears. Then, you move into the Cat Pose. Breathe out and move your stomach up toward your spine. Imagine a cat when it gets up from its nap and stretches its back. That is basically what you need to look like. Move your head toward the floor, but be careful not to put your chin into your chest. Breathe in, moving back into the Cow Pose, and then breathe out by moving into the Cat Pose. You can repeat this at least five times. When you need to come out of the poses, lift yourself up and sit back on your heels with your body in an upright position.

- **Forward Bending Pose:** This is one you can start by standing up. Basically, you bend over (forwards) and see if you can place your hands flat on the floor. Don't worry if you can't; don't force it and give yourself an injury. Just bend over as far as you can.

- **Relaxation Pose:** I'm sure you can guess what the benefit of this one is! Lie on the floor on your back with your hands by your sides, slightly outstretched, your palms facing up, and your legs slightly apart. Feel your body and feel the contact you have with the ground. Take a deep breath in. It's that simple.

Here's a yoga exercise for you to practice. Start with the grounding exercise I provided earlier. Then, once done, bring your hands up to be in front of your chest—almost as though you were saying a prayer. Breathe in, and then lift your arms up as high as you can. When you breathe out, drop your shoulders down—almost like you are shrugging. Repeat that: arms up/breathe in and shoulders down/breathe out four or five times. Then, when you reach up this time, put your palms together and look up if you can. Then, breathe out, let your hands come down to the "prayer" position, and put them down to where you had them in your grounding position.

MOVEMENT-BASED TECHNIQUES

As well as shaking practices and yoga, there are other techniques that involve somatic movement—that is, not so much worrying about what you look like while you are doing the movement but concentrating on what it feels like. Somatic movements are usually slow to give our bodies and brains a chance to learn them, performed with our complete concentration on our bodies' feelings and sensations. They usually have some purpose, whether physical or mental benefits or both.

These techniques include tense and release (conditioned) relaxation, where you tense and release each muscle in your body. These techniques should leave you feeling very chilled out and are easy to do whenever you want to anywhere in your house.

Here is a quick and simple tense and release exercise for you to practice. Please do be careful not to injure your muscles. If you get sharp pain at all, please stop.

Concentrate on a group of muscles; for instance, let's say your calf. Take a deep inhalation and tense that muscle until the point you feel some pressure on it; hold that for around five seconds. Then, you release while breathing out at the same time. It can be a good idea to visualize the muscle letting the tension out like air coming out of a burst tire or something similar—whatever works for you. Take note of the difference in how you and your body feel when relaxed compared to being tense. You should stay relaxed for approximately 10 seconds and then move on to the next muscle. Once you have completed all the muscle groups, relax, take in and enjoy the feeling of relaxation. All in all, it should take you 10 to 15 minutes to complete the exercise. The main muscle groups are your foot (curl your toes down), your calves, your thighs, your hands, your biceps, your butt, your stomach, your chest, your shoulders, your jaw, your eyes, and your forehead (raise your eyebrows).

You can also do this as a muscle relaxation exercise where you hold the tenseness for around 15 seconds and then let go and relax. For this, you just breathe normally—it doesn't matter when you inhale and exhale.

TRAUMA CLEARING SHAKING

Trauma clearing shaking exercises are designed to release the tension and trauma from the muscles deep inside your body. They involve a safe way of shaking that releases both tension from your muscles and calms your nervous system and you. You don't need a lot of time—maybe 20 minutes at most—and anybody can do it. It doesn't require you to be in any physical shape in particular. This very much ties in with the theory that the way animals cope with trauma is by "shaking it out," so to speak. When this safe way of shaking is engaged with, it suggests to the body that it returns to its normal balanced state. These types of exercises should leave you with a feeling of peace and tranquility.

For example: lie down on your back and place the soles of your feet together with your knees bent out. Then, raise your pelvis an inch or so off the floor and gradually pull your knees inward an inch or so every 30 seconds. After some time, you should reach a point where you begin to shake. If you are taking a long time to shake naturally, then this is because your muscles are very strong. You may need to hold the pose for longer. When ready, you can place the soles of your feet and pelvis on the ground and relax to let the trauma release through shaking. If you need to stop shaking, then you can just lengthen your legs out. Once you have finished, just lie down on your back and let yourself calm down and feel tranquil. It is quite a strange feeling to suddenly find your legs and body shaking, but that is what your body is designed to do when your muscles get fatigued, so it is all perfectly natural. It is very therapeutic as you shake out some of that trauma.

SOMATIC ART THERAPY

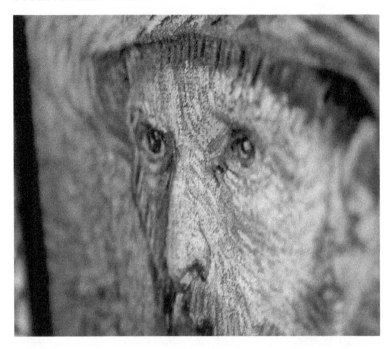

Don't worry. You don't have to be Van Gogh or Picasso to take part in art therapy, though they may have benefitted if they had done. Your art skills do not matter, but it is the therapeutic nature of it that matters. It is not just painting either; art means music, dance, sculpting, drawing, writing, and other art forms. The main point is that we learn about ourselves and our minds and bodies. It is not what your artistic finished product looks or sounds like. We know that we often express our innermost thoughts and feelings when we are creative. Look at any number of songwriters who deal with personal tragedy by writing a song about it. Look how we use someone else's art to express ourselves. I know there was a particular song I used to play which would help me grieve my mom's death. Playing it helped me break down, cry, and go through the grieving process. Without it, I had a stiff upper lip and kept everything inside, which, as we know, is rarely healthy.

It is said that because art engages our mental and physical capacities, it means we "forget" about whatever physical pain we may have. It is not simply something to take our mind off the pain, but it is something that relaxes us and, like some of the movement techniques, can set the body back to its normal state. Essentially, those suffering from severe chronic pain can greatly benefit from being involved in art therapy. A great study showed that 200 people in hospital either for surgery or a medical issue engaged in art therapy for 50 minutes. On average, they showed an improved mood and reduced their feelings of pain and anxiety (Shella, 2017).

We know that our soul, spirit, or psyche plays a huge part in our physical healing. That is why people will say "mind over matter" and the like. It is not your actual brain telling your body to be well, but the part of you that produces your feelings and thoughts. Art is the ultimate for expressing and engaging that subconscious part of ourselves, so it is no wonder it can help those who have constant pain—whether physical, psychological, or trauma-related. In this way, art therapy can be used alongside and in conjunction with traditional medicine to help people with any number of physical and mental health problems.

A quick art therapy exercise you can do is the following. Unfortunately, for art therapy, you need more than just yourself. For this, you need some crayons, coloring pencils, or pens. If you have paint, you may want to paint. You will also need some paper. Any paper will do—it doesn't need to be a special paper of any kind. Before you begin your art, just take some time to close your eyes and take a few deep breaths in and exhale with a longer breath. Just be in the moment and be aware of your body and what it is feeling and sensing. Once you feel ready, take your pen or pencil and draw a large circle on the paper. Now, inside the circle, draw how you are feeling at the moment. I know that's a hard thing to interpret, but go with what shapes and colors you are being pulled toward to represent your emotions. The circle represents a safe space, and therefore, you are free and able to express yourself within that circle. To learn what your drawing means, you can then do a writing exercise in which you ask the drawing questions, and the drawing, as though it were a person, can answer. Start off with some general questions and then work up to the specific questions about what the drawing's needs are and how the drawing intends to satisfy those needs. Don't feel like you have to follow a script; let the conversation go where you want it to go. Let whatever comes out of that dialogue just immerse itself into you. Don't try to force any conclusion or try to analyze what you have drawn and discussed. Just let it go into you, and by being in touch with your body and mind, what needs to happen or be addressed will work its way out in a natural way.

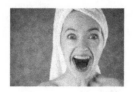

DO THESE PERSONALITIES
SOUND FAMILIAR?

During our lifetime, we will come into contact with a number of different people, all with their own unique identities and personalities. However, there are certain personalities that, if we come across them, are very capable of causing psychological damage and trauma. If we learn how to deal with these personalities and heal ourselves when we do come into contact—and it has an impact—then we could send our ability to self-love and self-compassion rocketing high. When we come into contact with these types of personalities, they cause us damage. It is not our fault: It is the other person who has the problem, not us. Unfortunately, they never resolve their problem, so we are often left with the weight of their unconsciousness as we try and recover from the trauma they cause. No more. After this chapter, you will be ready to forgive yourself and move on from past encounters with these personality types and be more prepared for when you come across them in the future.

NARCISSISTIC PERSONALITY DISORDER

This is quite a topical subject because there are commentators hinting that certain celebrities fit this personality type. All we have are rumors; none of us actually know the individuals in question, so it is a little bit much to point the finger. However, there are those who say that the reports of certain celebrities injuring staff, being aggressive toward staff, estranging family members from friends, and the need to give interviews about it all point to a classic narcissist. We're on the outside looking in, so we don't really know what is true and what is not, but it is an interesting premise.

Those that genuinely have a narcissistic personality disorder usually display an inflated sense of their own importance, a constant need for attention and respect, have problems showing any kind of empathy for other people, and most of the time, they have very difficult relationships. It can cause major issues in all areas of a person's life, such as their work, relationships, and financial stewardship. If someone with this disorder does not get the attention they need, they will be prone to becoming very unhappy and frustrated. Others will, more than likely, not enjoy their company and will steer clear.

Other signs of this disorder include wanting to be recognized as better than other people—even though they have not achieved anything to suggest that they are. They inflate their achievements and concentrate on illusions of grandeur about how powerful, rich, and beautiful they are. They may also exaggerate how they will find the perfect partner. Due to their own sense of superiority, they believe they can only socialize with those of equal or greater importance and will look down on anyone else. They will try to dominate conversations and often cut off or make sarcastic remarks toward those they consider not of the same standard. As they believe themselves to be higher than other people, they expect anyone inferior to treat them as such and that any such person would always be willing to answer any request. They may display signs of jealousy toward other people, and they would believe there are people who are jealous of them. They will always want the very best of every-thing—the best TV, best car, best phone, best house, and so on. Hence, the financial difficulties they can sometimes find themselves in.

Due to all of this, narcissists do not react well to any perceived criticism or suggestions on how they might want to improve their behavior. They can become very angry and frustrated if they do not receive the kind of compliant behavior they expect from other people. They will often get angry and try to put a person they see as inferior down, so they can feel better about themselves. In relation-ships, this type of behavior can end up as abuse—often psycholog-ical and sometimes even physical if the person cannot control their anger. You would never know where you stood with the person; the relationship would be the opposite of the safety and security you would be looking for. You can end up in a constant state of distress, wondering what is going to happen next and how your partner is going to behave or respond to anything and everything. If you do recognize these patterns of behavior in your relationships and believe you have suffered abuse as a result, please understand it was nothing about you that the abuser disliked or took exception to: They would have behaved that way to everybody. You may end up thinking there was something wrong with you. No, there was nothing wrong with you; they were the ones with the sickness. Don't feel like it was down to you to have tried to change their behavior. There really was nothing you could have done. They need to take responsibility for themselves.

It is not just in romantic relationships that narcissistic abuse can occur in; it can occur with members of your family or your colleagues or managers at work. Dealing with this type of disorder in those types of situations can also cause great trauma. Having a manager or colleague who sees you as inferior and expects you to happily meet their every demand can be exceptionally exhausting and demoralizing, to say the least. They are likely to fly off the handle at you if you do not comply with their demands. When it is a family member who you love, and they will not accept any criticism and do not have any empathy for you and your feelings, this can be heartbreaking. There is obviously plenty of opportunity for psychological damage that could take years to recover from, especially if this occurs when you are a young child.

Somatic therapy can be a helping hand to any narcissistic abuse. It is almost inevitable that with this kind of trauma, it does get stuck inside of you, and it is not something you are going to easily feel comfortable talking about. Therefore, just having talk therapy, though it may be helpful, is unlikely to get to the real crux of your trauma, whereas somatic therapy will be able to do that. It will help you release the trauma that is stuck deep inside of your body. This way, you can begin to heal. The boundary work we covered in a previous chapter can also be a great help should you find yourself in that kind of scenario ever again as, of course, is all the work on self-love, self-compassion, and self-forgiveness. None of this was your fault, and it is exceptionally important that you realize that and begin to love yourself again.

Another great method of helping to heal yourself from abuse is to take part in some EFT tapping. Tapping those vital energy fields and saying positive affirmations about what you went through and how you are going to heal from it can do wonders for the body and soul. Here is a short exercise for you to follow:

Inhale a deep breath and close your eyes. Make your body aware of the times in your past when you have come across narcissistic behavior. Maybe it is a situation that is occurring in the present. Take note of where in your body you are feeling the trauma. Inhale a deep breath and open your eyes.

- **1:** Start tapping the side of your hand. Say, "Despite the hurt and pain a narcissist has caused me, I still love and accept myself fully. A person in my past or in my present has caused me damage through their narcissism, and it is not easy to recover from that experience. I find it a struggle to move on and truly feel free from the pain. Despite the hurt and pain a narcissist has caused me, I still love, respect, and accept myself wholeheartedly. I hope the narcissist finds their own peace and manages to heal themselves and free themselves from their damaging behavior."

- **2:** Tap your forehead above your inner eyebrow, your temple, your cheekbone, your top lip, your chin, your heart area, under your armpit on the side of your ribs, and on the top of your head. Continue to repeat that cycle while saying the following:

The hurt, pain, and damage inflicted on me by narcissism. All the days, I was fearful because I did not know what to do or how to behave. I will heal from all of this. I may have been scared in the past to let myself heal. It was easier not to have to deal with the pain I was feeling and to believe that there was something wrong with me rather than with them. If I heal myself and love myself again, then it opens up the possibility of becoming hurt again in the future, so it is easier to do nothing. I love and accept those thoughts and feelings. Even though I know better now, they were natural thoughts and feelings. Now I am ready to heal myself from that experience.

I deserve to have calmness and serenity in my life. I deserve to love and be loved. The behavior shown to me was not actually about me, although that felt like the reality at the time. That's why it was so hard to let go of the hurt and pain, but I now know their behavior was not personal—it was just the symptoms of their sickness and not anything to do with me. I'm ready to heal. I am safe and secure. I am looking after myself. I have learned to set and respect boundaries. They belittled me and made me feel inferior, but I reject that notion. They are no better than me.

My life will not be dictated by this experience. Everything the person said was just their illness doing the speaking. It is not reality. I know the truth. I am an amazing person who is worthy of love and respect. I am ready to heal. I will heal. If someone truly loved and respected themselves, they would be able to love and respect me. People who are cruel to other people usually don't love and respect themselves to begin with. I acknowledge that, and I am moving on from that. I am healing from all that they have said and done. I love myself in ways that person never did, and other people will love me. I fully love and respect myself.

- **3:** Inhale a deep breath and close your eyes. Breathe out and open your eyes. Hopefully, those places in your body where you were feeling the trauma have now felt some relief, and you have let some of that tension and trauma go. Rinse and repeat as necessary.

Remember that it is okay and perfectly natural to be angry about this type of abuse. You were mistreated by partners, family, friends, or work colleagues. It was not due to anything you did: It was because they were sick. However, just because they were sick does not excuse what they did to you and what they put you through. You do not need to justify their behavior on their behalf. What they did was wrong—plain and simple. If you are angry about it, that is your right, and that is okay. Do not try to suppress your emotions or keep them bottled up inside of you, as that is not healthy. It is okay to be really angry at the person and what they did to you.

BORDERLINE PERSONALITY DISORDER

Borderline personality disorder will demonstrate itself in a person with wide-ranging moods and behavior. This will often result in some very impulsive decision-making and actions. BPD sufferers may have periods of severe anger, depression, or anxiety that can last several days.

The symptoms of this disorder can also include extreme mood swings and difficulty identifying with themselves and their place in the world. This means their likes and dislikes can change in an instant. They tend to see everything as one of two things: good or bad. This can make it difficult for those around them, as one day, they may think someone is their best friend, and the next day, they may believe them to be their worst enemy. Clearly, this can lead to some very unhealthy and volatile relationships with partners, friends, family, and work colleagues.

Those who have this illness may have issues of abandonment (whether they are real or not) and try to move relationships on too quickly or completely cut them off, so they are not the first to be abandoned. As mentioned in the first paragraph, impulsive behavior can be a result of borderline personality disorder. Therefore, the sufferer may go on expensive shopping outings, drive too quickly and without due care, have unprotected sexual relationships with many partners, may take to drugs or alcohol excessively, or even eat far too much in a short period of time. It is not unknown for sufferers to engage in self-harm or thoughts of suicide.

It can be the case that those that develop borderline personality disorder underwent traumatic events during their childhood, such as abuse or abandonment. Therefore, just as somatic therapy can heal those issues themselves, it can also help heal someone with borderline personality disorder. If we can heal the trauma within the person, that in turn should start to heal the mental illness. In addition, you can include CBT which will help a person be more aware of their thought patterns and how to change them. You can start to see how somatic therapy can help heal those with border-line personality disorder.

ABUSIVE PARTNERS IN RELATIONSHIPS

An abusive relationship can include physical or sexual abuse, emotional abuse, or neglect. Clearly, anyone who has to go through that kind of relationship with a person is not going to come out unscathed. It will more than likely cause trauma. It is likely to affect future behavior, and it may cause triggers so that ordinary things in life can cause a person to become fearful. The abuser may even cause you to doubt your own thoughts and feelings. They may have found a way to cut you off from your family and friends, so you no longer have anyone to tell you that your partner's behavior is wrong and you need to get out of the relationship. Once you've been through all of that, it makes it really difficult to ever trust anyone to be that close to you again.

In order to help you try to avoid ever getting involved in such relationships, these are the kinds of personalities and people you need to avoid. It is never easy, though, because part of the abuser's tool kit is to be able to charm you in those early stages of a relation-ship, only for their true colors to come out much later.

The most likely personality types to inflict abuse upon a person are the narcissist, which we have already covered, the sociopath, and the psychopath. Some of the character traits of all three can overlap.

Sociopaths tend not to be able to have empathy for anyone else, may indulge in impulsive behavior, will try to control other people usually in an aggressive manner, can be charming and charismatic, never learn from their mistakes or accept any punishment they may get for their behavior, will lie without a second thought, can often try to get into fights, may threaten harm to themselves without any intention of carrying it out, and may have issues with holding down a job or may get themselves into debt.

Psychopaths are not too dissimilar. As with a sociopath, psychopathy is not an actual psychiatric diagnosis. Someone who aligns with these traits may actually be diagnosed as having antisocial personality disorder (ASPD). The antisocial aspect comes not from them being unsociable—as like sociopaths, they are capable of great charm and charisma—but from their tendency to not care too much for the rules of society (Lindberg, 2019). As well as not being too concerned with society, they are not going to be concerned about anybody else's safety or well-being. They will not have much of a moral compass, they will be a consistent liar, and they may engage in very reckless and dangerous behavior. They are more than likely to demonstrate great anger and generally be quite aggressive.

Somatic therapy can be a healer for anyone who is going through or has come out of an abusive relationship. It really can lessen those emotional scars. It can ease the trauma out of your body in a safe and secure way. It can help you get to know yourself again, realize the truth of the situation—that it was not your fault —and help to love yourself again and to forgive yourself.

Let's do a quick exercise that will start you on your way to healing from an abusive relationship. Sit comfortably and close your eyes. Be aware of what your body feels when you remember this abusive relationship. Take note of what it feels. Practice your deep breathing, and as you are doing this, say the following: "I am accepting of this feeling. I love myself. I am healing myself. I was fearful, but now I am safe and secure. I want to heal, and I know I can heal." Just keep breathing and saying these sentences, and you should start to feel your body heal over time.

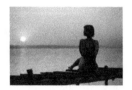

WHERE TO GO FROM HERE—
HOW TO KNOW YOU'RE HEALING

It's one thing to take part in somatic therapy, but how do you know it's working? That's what this chapter is all about—knowing when you are healing. You will be able to spot the signs that tell you the healing is taking place. It will make it clear to you how to tell what you have achieved thus far and what you still need to work on and improve. It also helps to manage your expectations in terms of how long it may take you to fully heal and recover. The main thing to remember above all is that even if you are finding it difficult to heal and love yourself at this moment in time, you are not alone. I have been through some of the experiences in this book, so I want you to know that you have my support, love, and respect. It's all wrapped up in the words on these pages—hopefully as a constant source of comfort to you. It's also always wise to seek outside support from others that may have been through what you have.

HOW TO KNOW WHEN YOU ARE HEALING

One thing to bear in mind is that healing is not something that is going to occur after just two minutes of breathing practice. It is something you have to adopt as a major part of your life in order to achieve. It's not like a broken leg—you wrap it in plaster, leave it alone, and it heals—that's it. No, you have to keep on practicing somatic therapy and really integrate it into your life for it to be a complete success.

So how do you tell the therapy is working? First of all, it'll show through your nervous system, which as you go through therapy should become much more regulated and much more in harmony. Your fight-or-flight response should be becoming more settled, and your heart rate should be at a normal rate. You should be sleeping well, and your digestion should be good. Your immune system should be stronger. Your blood pressure should be normal. Of course, not all of these things are going to change overnight. If you were having specific issues in any of those areas, over time, you should start seeing minor improvements. Maybe you noticed you slept a bit better, or you are able to go to the restroom on a more regular basis. This isn't just the physical side of things either— maybe you notice you were able to set a boundary whereas before, that would have scared you greatly. Whatever it may be, you should see those slight changes occur the more you do the work.

The other way you may notice a difference is in your ability to let more into your life. When the trauma is stuck in your body, and it is having all these negative effects on your life, you find you don't really do a lot, and you don't really want to have too many people in your life, as you are anxious or stressed about so many situations and people. It could be that something triggered you, and you go into retreat. Or something happens, and you get angry and can't calm down from it. When you are healing, you start noticing that you can take more on. Fewer things make you anxious and stress you out, so you have more time to spend actually living life. Whereas you were getting angry and couldn't calm down, now things are happening. It's like water off a duck's back: You just get on with it.

Those are the two main ways you can monitor and notice

whether the healing is working. If you're reading this after conducting somatic therapy for a while and you are noticing some of those improvements, well done! You are healing, and may you continue to heal. If you are just at the beginning of the journey, you can now look forward to spotting these types of improvements over time so that you can live life to the fullest and be the best version of yourself that you possibly can. I look forward to seeing you achieve that as well.

WHAT TO LOOK FOR IN A SOMATIC THERAPIST

Although we have concentrated on exercises you can do at home, to truly have access to everything involved in somatic therapy, you are probably going to want to find a somatic therapist. You might want to review the therapist's qualifications, experience, and whether they are licensed: If they aren't, cross them off your list.

With a therapist, you have the added indicator that you need to feel comfortable with them. You need to feel that they understand you, and they are in agreement with the issues you are looking to address. One way to fathom this out is to ask the very simple question of whether they can help you. From their response, you should get a good feel for whether you are going to be comfortable with them. You can always ask some follow-up questions as well. I would hope this book has given some confidence and plenty of knowledge to have the confidence to ask those questions. You are probably going to want to ask what their plan of action is: What exactly is the treatment they are likely to be recommending for you? This will help give you a really good idea of whether this is someone you can trust. Have they understood you and based on your trauma be able to apply a rough plan for you? Equally, are they big enough to admit that things may change as you go along? As things come up in sessions, they may need to adapt their plan. It's good to know if they are humble enough to admit that is a possibility. Equally, don't trust someone who says following their plan will definitely heal you in a specific amount of time. They don't really know how things can turn out. They may have a good idea, but no one can know for sure until you start doing the work. Therapists making definite promises are probably not to be trusted. Based on all of this, you probably don't want to find a therapist who is going to make you commit to a long period of therapy for a huge amount of money, given that any plan made for this type of thing could well change. You want them to be as adaptable and flexible in their outlook as possible.

It's not just about feeling comfortable as well: It's about whether you actually like the person. You could imagine them as someone whose company you like to be in. In a sense, one way leads to the other, as you are unlikely to ever feel comfortable in the presence of someone you didn't like. However, it's not just about being comfortable, particularly as having been through trauma, you may not feel comfortable with yourself, let alone anyone else. Start to use that somatic sense already, and see whether you feel you like the therapist as a person or not.

When it comes to qualifications, at the very least, you are going to want a therapist who has had training in somatic experiencing. Ideally, you probably want them to be qualified with something else —a slightly different field to somatic experiencing so that they aren't just focused on the one way to do things. It's always nice to see someone who is progressing as well. They haven't just trained at one thing and stopped: They have continued to learn and grow as a therapist. One of the biggest qualifications can be if they have done the work on themselves and if they used their own somatic therapy to heal themselves. It suggests what they did worked, and they should have some experience of what you have been through. Ultimately, they should be able to understand and have empathy for you.

Remember that as long as you haven't signed some dodgy contract that states you can never leave, you don't have to do anything. If, after a while, you feel it isn't really working for you, then there is nothing to stop you from ending the therapy there.

You are never under pressure to have to stay doing something that is making no difference to you. You can always seek out alternative therapists and alternative therapies.

FINDING MEANING AFTER TRAUMA

It can be hard when you've been through trauma, even if you are healing or have begun to heal. You know you want to move on, but you don't know where you want to move on. Below are some tips to assist you in finding yourself and finding meaning after trauma.

One tip is to try and lead a fulfilling life. I know that's easier said than done, but after everything you've been through, you probably feel like there is a big hole in your life. What do you want to fill it with? Think about what it is you want that means you look forward to waking up tomorrow and seizing the day.

If there are things stopping you from fulfilling your life, then it's time to admit they exist—not as a bad thing or as something to feel guilty about but in a pragmatic, accepting way. All this trauma has actually caused me to be, let's say, "distant" in relationships. Now, I accept that it is the case, and this is now an opportunity for me to slowly change that. It may be painful, and it may be difficult, but if we can accept there may be things that stop us from progressing, rather than see them as a negative, we can see it as a chance to try better this time and turn it into an opportunity.

An important thing to remember is that by getting through this and still being here, you are an exceptionally resilient person. That means you can probably get through anything. You are a strong person, even if it sometimes doesn't feel like it, and that really is an important lesson you have learned. Through your somatic therapy, you will only grow even further as a person. Although what you went through was terrible, and you would much rather have never gone through it, it will have made you stronger in the long run. This is a way of saying, also, that we need to find meaning in life. Without that meaning, we usually drift along without knowing where we are going. It's important to do the things and see the people that bring meaning to your life. If you can do that, then you can fill the hole that trauma has left you.

THE SOMATIC DAILY RITUAL FOR EMPOWERED HEALING

Throughout the chapters, I've tried to give you some examples and exercises to work on and see what impact they have. However, the best thing is to bring much of that together into one daily ritual to get an enhanced healing experience. I've included aspects from various chapters in this book. All in all, the ritual should take you around 30 minutes, so you should still be able to fit this into your day. I think this ritual works particularly well in the morning, as it has elements of both releasing tension and relaxing you but also getting you ready to face the day ahead.

Once you've got the hang of this one, you can easily write your own ritual with the knowledge and experience you have built up. You can even put it up on your wall or fridge for that constant reminder and inspiration for you to complete it each day.

1: BREATH WORK (FIVE MINUTES):

- Find a comfortable place to sit. You don't need to sit up completely straight, but your back does need to be supported.
- Close your eyes.
- Take three deep breaths: Inhale through the nose and exhale through the mouth.
- Put one hand on your belly and one hand on your chest. Take 10 deep breaths. You should be able to feel the air start off in your belly and work its way up toward and into your chest.

- Take 10 deep breaths: inhale and exhale out of the nose.
- Take 10 deep breaths: inhale out of the nose and exhale out of the mouth.
- Take 10 deep breaths: Inhale and exhale out of the mouth.
- Inhale one last deep breath. Hold it for seven seconds. Exhale and relax.
- Relax for 30 seconds, breathing normally.
- Open your eyes.

2: Mindfulness Exercise (Five Minutes):

- Make sure you are in a comfortable position.
- Close your eyes.
- Become aware of your body, and see if there are any specific areas that feel relaxed. Focus on one part of your body that is feeling good and relaxed. Concentrate on that one place and the feeling.
- Think of a word that best describes this feeling.
- Take note of any changes to your breath when focusing on the relaxed and happy places in your body.
- To end the exercise, start to slowly take note of the sounds and smells around you.
- When you are ready, open your eyes.

3: EFT Tapping (Five Minutes):

- The cycle will include tapping on the side of your hand for a minute, followed by a continual cycle of the top of the head, inner forehead above the right eyebrow, temple, cheekbone, top lip, chin, heart area, and under the armpit on the side of your ribs.
- Say the following while tapping: "I love and accept myself wholeheartedly. I am ready to heal. I found it

difficult in the past to accept the truth or that I had done nothing wrong and that I am a good person. I now know that to be true. I can't forget my past, but I can move on from it. I accept myself for who I am. I am a beautiful, loving human being, and I deserve to be loved. I respect and accept myself. I am ready to heal, and I will heal."

- Take your time doing the tapping. You do not need to rush from one stage to the next. Take your time saying the affirmations. You can choose not to say them if you don't feel they apply or add in anything you feel to be more appropriate.

4: Qigong (Five Minutes):

- Take a standing position. Make sure you are nicely relaxed and stand with your feet slightly apart.
- Take a breath in and reach up with your hands.
- Breathe out and bring your hands down to the center of your body. Have your hands facing each other with palms down—almost like you are pushing something down with the air below the hands.
- Rub your hands together like you are trying to start a fire with them until they start to feel warm.
- Once they are warm, close your eyes and place the palm of your hands on your eyelids. Keep them on there for approximately 30 seconds.
- Take your hands away from your eyelids and rub them all over your face. Rub your face 10 to 30 times.
- Now, stroke your fingers through your hair. This is dependent on how much hair you have. It may just be a short run, or you may be able to run your fingers through your hair for quite some time. Do this 10 to 30 times, depending on how much time you have to spare.

- Rub your ears. You are basically giving your ears a massage, so you can rub your ears or pull your ears—whatever feels good to you.
- Put your hands gently on your neck and press on the muscles. Gently is key: You don't want to give yourself an injury.
- Find the part of your spine that sticks out just below your shoulders. Gently tap it with one hand, then tap it with the other hand. Do this for five seconds with each hand.
- If you are still feeling any tension after that, just do a quick shake of your whole body. As you have been using your arms a lot, particularly shake off the tension from your hands, arms, and shoulders.
- End with breathing in, reaching up, and breathing out—bringing your hands down.

5: Somatic Yoga Exercise (10 Minutes):

- Start with a Forward Bend Pose.
- Move slowly into a Standing Cat-Cow Pose with your knees bent, moving your hands up to your knees and gently raising your back and head.
- Go back into the Forward Bend Pose and repeat, going into the Standing Cat-Cow Pose and back to the Forward Bend Pose a couple of times.
- Move into a standing position crouched over, but put your elbows into the top of your thighs and gently and slowly move your elbows down your thighs until you reach your knees. Do this three or four times.
- Do the Standing Cat-Cow Pose with your knees bent. Moving from a Cow Pose to a Cat Pose. Do this five times.
- Stand with your legs apart and swish your arms from one

side to the other, one arm at a time. Start off slowly and speed up the movement. Do this five times.

- Do the Standing Cat-Cow Pose on your hands and knees. Do this five times.
- Go into Child's Pose. Hold it for a few moments.
- Go on your back with your arms outstretched behind you. Swing your leg over from one side to the other. Do the same for the other leg. Do this five times.
- Stay on your back and put the soles of your feet together with your knees bent. Hold this for a few moments.
- Pull yourself up to sit cross-legged with your arms resting on your legs. Hold it for a few moments.

AFTERWORD

Well done! I wish you incredible power on your somatic adventure. You've made it through to the end. That in itself is something to be proud of. You can congratulate yourself for taking that first step in becoming curious about somatic therapy and reading about it. I am confident that with your curiosity, combined with the advice and practices in this book, you will be well on the way to healing from the trauma you have undergone in the past. Just reading this book shows your bravery in wanting to heal from the trauma, and you will need that bravery as you continue on your journey.

Trauma is an all-encompassing event that we go through. For so long, people have surmised that it is something that only happens in the brain. Now we know so much more—that it happens in the brain, the body, and the spirit. One of the only ways to reach all those three things and truly heal is from somatic therapy. I'm not saying "talk therapy" isn't useful because, of course, it can be. Still, talk therapy alone won't always get to the root of the trauma in your body, and, sometimes, talk therapy can be the worst thing for someone with trauma to go through as they are going to be asked to bring up their traumatic experiences. There is little titration practiced in talk therapy, but working with somatic therapy helps you release that trauma little by little—not just through talking and using your mind but by becoming in touch with and aware of what your body feels and senses.

The trouble with trauma is that it also ends up causing other issues such as chronic pain, depression, anxiety, addiction, digestion issues, and lack of sleep, but all these things can be addressed and worked through with somatic therapy. Another wonderful thing about somatic therapy is that there are so many elements that you are not stuck with just doing one method or another; there are a variety of techniques and exercises that can be employed. Sometimes, it can be trial and error, but you should find something that suits you and works for you.

Through the concepts that somatic therapy teaches us, we really gain an understanding of our body, how it works, and how we can best get it to work for us. Grounding is a great exercise for just getting yourself settled and becoming aware of your body and what it is feeling. If ever you find your mind is racing away with you or you are becoming a bit panicked or anxious, one of the best things to do is to take a few moments to sit down with your feet firmly on the floor and go through some grounding techniques. I nearly always feel calmer and more at peace having done that and gotten in touch with my body and listened to it. It's almost like my body thanks me for listening to it.

Setting and maintaining boundaries can be an essential exercise for many—particularly those who have submerged themselves into others' lives or those that have been in abusive relationships. It also helps to keep things in the present and the here and now, which is where we all want to live.

As I touched upon in the last chapter, going through somatic therapy helps you start to self-regulate your nervous system, and over the long term, this can have such an important impact. Your emotions are self-regulated. No longer do you get upset at someone for seemingly no reason. Well, I'm not saying ever: We all get tired and grumpy sometimes but not because you have trauma that is still trapped in your body. Your fight-or-flight response becomes more regulated, so not every single thing will send you into a state of panic and anxiety. Slowly, your decision-making process becomes more in line with what it should be. Your digestion, sleep, and so many things can become more regulated, and all of it leads to your recovery, healing, and having the kind of life you imagine having for yourself. Self-regulation is such a vital part and goal of somatic therapy.

The use of movement can also be considered a cornerstone of the somatic experience. This doesn't have to be dance (though that is available in art therapy) or anything overly energetic. It can be as simple as a few postures in yoga, some shaking in Qigong, or some muscle tensing and releasing. These can be as energetic as you want or as serene as you want, but that movement is another part of getting to know your body, being aware of your body, and listening to what it is saying to you. All of these movements address the fact that trauma is in your body—not just in your mind.

There is no doubt in my mind that you have made the right decision. Somatic therapy is one of the best ways for you to heal yourself from your trauma. I'm proud of you for taking such a monumental step. I wish I could be there with you by your side as you go through your somatic journey, but hopefully, you feel I am there with you, cheering you on in the form of this book. You can transform your life and lead a life so much less full of pain and hurt than is currently the situation. You can start to look forward to life. You can start to be excited to wake up in the morning—not wake up with that horrible feeling of dread in the pit of your stomach. You actually can't wait to see what the day has in store for you.

You are no longer controlled by the trauma, and you have taken control of your life. This is such a powerful statement and one that will be true. You have the rest of your life to live; go and enjoy it.

It's so easy to incorporate so much of this into your daily routine as well. Even the ritual I provide only takes 30 minutes out of your day. So much of it can be done when you wake up or just before you go to bed that you can easily make sure you accomplish it. All you need is a quiet space in your house (sometimes easier said than done, I know), and away you go.

This is your body. This is your life. Go and make it the best it can possibly be. All the best and, as the whole of this book encourages you to, take care of yourself.

REFERENCES

All images are courtesy of Pixabay.

Barnes, S., Brown, K., Krusemark, E., Campbell, W & Rogge, R. (2007, October 11). *The Role of Mindfulness in Romantic Relationship Satisfaction and Responses to Relationship Stress.* Journal of Family and Marital Therapy. https://doi.org/10.1111/j.1752-0606.2007.00033.x

Baxter, S. (2019, October 20). *Vagus Nerve Reset to Release Trauma Stored in the Body (Polyvagal Exercises).* Vagus Nerve Reset To Release Trauma Stored In The Body (Polyvagal Exercises) - YouTube

Baxter, S. (2020, November 9). *Vagus Nerve Exercises to Rewire Your Brain from Anxiety.* Vagus Nerve Exercises To Rewire Your Brain From Anxiety - YouTube

Bell, A. (2017, July 21). *Somatic Psychotherapy.* Good Therapy. Somatic Psychotherapy (goodtherapy.org)

Bell, A. (2018, June 19). *Somatic Mindfulness: What Is My Body Telling Me? (And Should I Listen?).* Good Therapy. https://www.goodthera-py.org/blog/somatic-mindfulness-what-is-my-body-telling-me-and-should-i-listen-0619185

Brom, D., Stokar, Y., Lawi, C., Nuriel-Porat, V., Ziv, Y., Lerner, K. & Ross, G. (2017, June 6). *Somatic Experiencing for Posttraumatic Stress*

Disorder: A Randomized Controlled Outcome Study. Wiley Online
Library. https://dx.doi.org/10.1002%2Fjts.22189

Butler, A., Chapman, J., Forman, E & Beck, A. (2006, January). *The
Empirical Status of Cognitive-Behavioral Therapy: A Review of Meta-
Analyses.* Clinical Psychology Review. https://psycnet.a-
pa.org/doi/10.1016/j.cpr.2005.07.003

Carbonelli, D. & Parteleno-Barehmi, C. (2016, May 11). *Psychodrama
Groups for Girls Coping With Trauma.* Taylor & Francis Online.
https://doi.org/10.1080/00207284.1999.11732607

Chambers, R., Chuen Yee Lo, B. & Allen, N. (2007, February 23).
*The Impact of Intensive Mindfulness and Training on Attention Control,
Cognitive Style, and Affect.* Springer Link.
http://dx.doi.org/10.1007/s10608-007-9119-0

Chen, Y., Hung, K., Tsai, J., Chu, H., Chung, M., Chen, S., Liao, Y.,
Ou, K., Chang, Y. & Chou, K. (2014, August 7). *Efficacy of Eye-
Movement Desensitization and Reprocessing for Patients with
Posttraumatic-Stress Disorder: A Meta-Analysis of Randomized Controlled
Trials.* PLOS ONE.
https://dx.doi.org/10.1371%2Fjournal.pone.0103676

Cino, R. (2017, November 24). *How to Decrease Anxiety Using Somatic
Experiencing.* myTherapyNYC. https://mytherapynyc.com/how-to-
decrease-anxiety-using-somatic-experiencing/#comments

Clarke, J. (2021, July 31). *What Is Gestalt Therapy?* Verywell Mind.
https://www.verywellmind.com/what-is-gestalt-therapy-4584583

ConciousnessNOWTV. (2020, September 19). *How to use
Pendulation to Decrease Stress and Increase Well-Being.* How to use
Pendulation to Decrease Stress and Increase Well-Being - YouTube

Counselling and Meditation Exercises. (n.d.) Sligo Gestalt Counselling.
https://sligogestaltcounselling.ie/try-these-counselling-
exercises.html

Cutler, N. (n.d.) *Learning How to Unlock Tissue Memory.* Integrated
Physical Therapy and Wellness.
https://www.iptmiami.com/news/Learning_How_to_Unlock_Tis-
sue_Memory

Depressive Disorders. (n.d.) Psychology Today. https://www.psychologytoday.com/us/conditions/depressive-disorders

Diaphragmatic Breathing Exercises. (n.d.). Physiopedia. https://www.physio-pedia.com/Diaphragmatic_Breathing_Exercises

Diaphragmatic Breathing: Everything You Need to Know. (n.d.). Evolve Chiropractic. https://myevolvechiropractor.com/diaphragmatic-breathing/

Eckelkamp, S. (2019, October 9). *Can Trauma Really be 'Stored' in the Body?* mbg Health. https://www.mindbodygreen.com/articles/can-trauma-be-stored-in-body

Energy Psychology (2017, October 26). Good Psychology. https://www.goodtherapy.org/learn-about-therapy/types/energy-psychology

Erdelyi, K. (2019, October 28). *What is Somatic Therapy?* Psycom. https://www.psycom.net/what-is-somatic-therapy/

Essential Somatics. (2019, February 1). *The Best Psoas Release.* (2) The Best Psoas Release - YouTube

Fallis, J. (2021, March 24). *How to Stimulate Your Vagus Nerve for Better Mental Health.* Optimal Living Dynamics. https://www.optimallivingdynamics.com/blog/how-to-stimulate-your-vagus-nerve-for-better-mental-health-brain-vns-ways-treatment-activate-natural-foods-depression-anxiety-stress-heart-rate-variability-yoga-massage-vagal-tone-dysfunction

Feinstein, D. (2012, December 1). *Acupoint Stimulation in Treating Psychological Disorders: Evidence of Efficacy.* Sage Journals. https://doi.org/10.1037%2Fa0028602

Field, T. & Diego, M. (2008, March 4). *Vagal Activity, Early Growth and Emotional Development.* PubMed Central. https://dx.doi.org/10.1016%2Fj.infbeh.2007.12.008

Forgiveness: Your Health Depends On It. (n.d.) John Hopkins Medicine. https://www.hopkinsmedicine.org/health/wellness-and-prevention/forgiveness-your-health-depends-on-it

Friedman, L. (2019, November 15). *Using Somatic Experiencing to Cope with Anger.* Trauma & Beyond. Using Somatic Experiencing to Cope with Anger | Trauma Therapy (traumaandbeyondcenter.com)

Gaba, S. (2020, August 22). *Understanding Fight, Flight, Freeze and the Fawn Response.* Psychology Today. https://www.psychologytoday.com/gb/blog/addiction-and-recovery/202008/understanding-fight-flight-freeze-and-the-fawn-response

Giacomucci, S. & Marquit, J. (2020, May 19). *The Effectiveness of Trauma-Focused Psychodrama in the Treatment of PTSD in Inpatient Substance Abuse Treatment.* Frontiers in Psychology. https://doi.org/10.3389/fpsyg.2020.00896

Goodlet, N. (2020, November 30). *Vagus Nerve Stimulation Breathing Meditation Practice.* https://www.youtube.com/watch?v=kiQMaJJWcyQ

Hadley, H. (2017, July 19). *The Benefits of Somatic Breathing.* Total Somatics. https://totalsomatics.com/the-benefits-of-somatic-breathing/

Heidari, S., Shahbakhsh, B. & Jangjoo, M. (2017). *The Effectiveness of Gestalt Therapy on Depressed Women in Comparison with Drug Therapy.* Journal of Applied Psychology and Behavioral Science. https://japbs.com/fulltext/paper-02012017134122.pdf

Hoffman, S., Sawyer, A., Witt. A & Oh, D. (2010, April 1). *The Effect of Mindfulness-Based Therapy on Anxiety and Depression: A Meta-Analytic Review.* PMC. https://www.ncbi.nlm.nih.gov/pmc/articles/PMC2848393/

Holmes, J. & McGauran, J. (Executive Producers). (1988–present). *Home and Away* [TV series]. Seven Studios; Seven Network Operations Limited; Red Heart Entertainment; Keeper Media.

Hopper, S., Murray, S., Ferrara, L. & Singleton, J. (2019, September). *Effectiveness of Diaphragmatic Breathing for Reducing Physiological and Psychological Stress in Adults: A Quantitative Systematic Review.* JBI Evidence Synthesis. https://doi.org/10.11124/jbisrir-2017-003848

IABET - Consciousness Through Art. (2020, April 2). *Art Therapy Exercise - Exploring Emotional Needs.* Art Therapy Exercise - Exploring Emotional Needs - YouTube

Jackson, K. (2019, February 4). *Pandiculations 101 with Think Somatics.* (2) Pandiculations 101 with Think Somatics - YouTube

Jackson, T. (2017, August 24). *Grounding: What to Do When You Feel Unstable*. Toni Jackson Counselling. https://tonijacksoncoun-selling.com/2017/08/24/grounding-what-to-do-when-you-feel-unstable/

Jahnke, R., Larkey, L., Rogers, C., Etnier, J. & Lin, F. (2010, July 1). *A Comprehensive Review of Health Benefits of Qigong and Tai Chi*. Sage Journals. https://journals.sagepub.com/doi/10.4278/ajhp.081013-LIT-248?url_ver=Z39.88-2003&rfr_id=ori%3Arid%3Acrossre-f.org&rfr_dat=cr_pub%3Dpubmed&

Janet, S. & Gowri, P. (2017). *Effectiveness of Deep Breathing Exercise on Blood Pressure Among Patients with Hypertension*. International Journal of Pharma and Bio Science. http://dx.doi.org/10.22376/ijpbs.2017.8.1.b256-260

Jerath, R., Beveridge, C. & Barnes, V. (2019, January 29). *Self-Regulation Breathing of Breathing as an Adjunctive Treatment of Insomnia*. Frontiers. https://doi.org/10.3389/fpsyt.2018.00780

Johnson, J. (2020. May 27). *What to Know About Diaphragmatic Breathing*. Medical News Today. What is diaphragmatic breathing? Benefits and how-to (medicalnewstoday.com)

Jordan, S. (2016, February 7). *An Introduction to Focusing*. British Focusing Association. https://www.focusing.org.uk/an-introduction-to-focusing

Kelloway, R. (2019, March 29). *5 Somatic Experiencing Exercises to Keep Grounded During Coronavirus Uncertainty*. Life Care Wellness. https://life-care-wellness.com/somatic-experiencing-exercises-to-keep-you-grounded/

KoK, B., Coffey, K. & Cohn, M. (2013, May 6). *How Positive Emotions Build Physical Health: Perceived Positive Social Connections Account for the Upward Spiral Between Positive Emotions and Vagal Tone*. Sage Journals. https://doi.org/10.1177%2F0956797612470827

Langmuir, J., Kirsch, S. & Classen, C. (2012). *A Pilot Study of Body-Orientated Group Psychotherapy for the Group Treatment of Trauma*. APA PsycNet. https://psycnet.apa.org/doi/10.1037/a0025588

Leung, G & Khor, S. (2017, April 25). *Gestalt Intervention Groups for*

Anxious Parents in Hong Kong: A Quasi-Experimental Design. Taylor & Francis Online. https://doi.org/10.1080/23761407.2017.1311814

Lindberg, S. (2019, January 9). *Psychopath.* Healthline. https://www.healthline.com/health/psychopath

Lynch, D., Laws, K & McKenna, P. (2009, May 29). *Cognitive Behavioral Therapy for Major Psychiatric Disorder: Does It Really Work? A Meta-Analytical Review of Well-Controlled Trials.* Cambridge University Press. https://doi.org/10.1017/s003329170900590x

Lyon, B. (2017, August 1). *Shame and Trauma.* Center for Healing Shame. https://healingshame.com/articles/2017/8/21/shame-and-trauma

Ma, X., Yue, Z., Gong, Z., Zhang, H., Duan, N., Shi, Y., Wei. G. & Li, Y. (2017, June 6). *The Effect of Diaphragmatic Breathing on Attention, Negative Affect and Stress in Healthy Adults.* PubMed Central. https://dx.doi.org/10.3389%2Ffpsyg.2017.00874

MacCarthy, M. (2019, December 17). *Somatic Low Back & Psoas Release.* (2) Somatic Low Back & Psoas Release - YouTube

Mertz, C. (2013). *The Effectiveness of Psychodrama for Adolescents who have Experienced Trauma.* Smith ScholarWorks. https://scholarworks.smith.edu/cgi/viewcontent.cgi?article=2024&context=theses

Meyer, A. (2020, June 20). *Subconscious Mind & Inner Child Explained: The Key to Wellbeing.* Medium. https://medium.com/invisible-illness/the-subconscious-mind-inner-child-explained-511b1ef93c7f

Miller, B., Littlefield, W., Morano, R., Wilson, D., Sears, F., Chaiken, I., Moss, E., Barker, M., Tuchman, E., Chang, Y., Hockin, S., Weber, J., Siracusa, F., & Fortenberry, D. (Executive Producers). (2017–present). *The Handmaid's Tale* [TV series]. Daniel Wilson Productions Inc.; The Littlefield Company; White Oak Pictures; MGM Studios.

Millman, R. (2019, March 24). *Healing the Inner Child | Tapping with Renee.* Healing The Inner Child | Tapping with Renee - YouTube

Millman, R. (2020, February 16). *Tapping to Heal the Inner Child and Letting Go of Shame | Tapping with Renee.* Tapping To Heal The Inner Child and Letting Go Of Shame | Tapping With Renee - YouTube

Moore, A. & Malinowski, P. (2009, March 18). *Meditation, Mindfulness and Cognitive Flexibility.* PubMed. https://pubmed.ncbi.nlm.nih.gov/19181542/

Morrisey, S. & Marr, J. (1984). Still Ill (Song) on *The Smiths.* Rough Trade.

Ortner, C., Kilner, S. & Zelazo, P. (2007, November 20). *Mindfulness Meditation and Reduced Emotional Interference on a Cognitive Task.* Springer Link. https://link.springer.com/article/10.1007/s11031-007-9076-7

Osadchey, S. (2028, August 8). *Somatic Experiencing (SE).* Good Therapy. https://www.goodtherapy.org/learn-about-therapy/types/somatic-experiencing

Pandiculation - The Safe Alternative to Stretching. (2010, September 30). Essential Somatics. https://essentialsomatics.com/clinical-somatics-articles-case-studies/pandiculation-safe-alternative-stretching

Psychodrama. (2016, May 16). Good Therapy. https://www.goodtherapy.org/learn-about-therapy/types/psychodrama

Richmond, C. (2018, November 29). *Emotional Trauma and the Mind-Body Connection.* WebMD. https://www.webmd.com/mental-health/features/emotional-trauma-mind-body-connection

Saadati, H. & Lashani, L. (2013, July 9). *Effectiveness of Gestalt Therapy on Self-Efficacy of Divorced Women.* Science Direct. https://doi.org/10.1016/j.sbspro.2013.06.721

Sensorimotor Psychotherapy. (2015, August 24). Good Therapy. Sensorimotor Psychotherapy (goodtherapy.org)

Shapiro, F. (2014). *The Role of Eye Movement Desensitization and Reprocessing (EMDR) Therapy in Medicine: Addressing the Psychological and Physical Symptoms Stemming from Adverse Life Experience.* The Permanente Journal. https://dx.doi.org/10.7812%2FTPP%2F13-098

Shella. T. (2017, May 26). *Art Therapy Improves Mood, and Reduces Pain and Anxiety When Offered at Bedside During Acute Hospital Treatment.* Science Direct. https://www.sciencedirect.com/science/article/abs/pii/S0197455617301053

Somatic Experiencing International. (2019, August 15). *What is*

Pendulation in Somatic Experiencing with Peter A Levine, PhD. https://www.youtube.com/watch?v=LiXOMLoDm68&t=1s

Tomasulo, D. (2021, June 18). *Do You Need a Mama Psychodrama?* LinkedIn. https://www.linkedin.com/pulse/do-you-need-mama-psychodrama-dan-tomasulo

Transformations Treatment Center. (2018, October 1). *EMDR: Self-Soothing at Home. (2) EMDR: Self-soothing at home - YouTube*

Tune Up Fitness (2020, March 10). *Hum to Activate the Vagus Nerve.* Hum to Activate the Vagus Nerve - YouTube

Tune Up Fitness. (2020, March 10). *Vagus Nerve: Breathing for Relaxation.* Vagus Nerve: Breathing for Relaxation - YouTube

Valiente-Gomez, A., Moreno-Alcazar, A., Treen, D., Cedron, C., Colom, F., Perez, V. & Amann, B. (2017, September 26). *EMDR Beyond PTSD: A Systematic Literature Review.* Frontiers in Psychology. https://doi.org/10.3389/fpsyg.2017.01668

Van Korff, M., Crane, P., Lane, M., Miglioretti, D., Simon, G., Saunders, K., Stang, P., Brandenburg, N. & Kessler, R. (2005, February). *Chronic Spinal Pain and Physical-Mental Comorobidiy in the United States: Results From the National Comorbidity Survey Replication.* PAIN 10.1016/j.pain.2004.11.010

Virant, K. (2019, May 12). *Chronic Illness and Trauma Disorders.* Psychology Today. https://www.psychologytoday.com/gb/blog/chronically-me/201905/chronic-illness-and-trauma-disorders

Wagner, D. (2016, June 27). *Polyvagal Theory in Practice.* Counseling Today. Polyvagal theory in practice - Counseling Today

Warren, S. (2019, April 21). *What is Pandiculation?* Somatic Movement Center. https://somaticmovementcenter.com/pandiculation-what-is-pandiculation/

Winn, A. (2019, August 15). *Energy Psychology Demonstration - Correct Demo of Cooks Hook Up.* (3) Energy psychology demonstration - Correct demo of Cooks Hookup - YouTube

Yates, B. (2013, September 28). *Self-Love in About Five Minutes -*

Tapping with Brad Yates. https://www.youtube.com/watch?v=tLWTzQWa2hg

Yates, B. (2014, February 28). *Self-Compassion - Tapping with Brad Yates.* https://www.youtube.com/watch?v=KHydpkmWydI

Yates, B. (2020, August 31). *Narcissists (Getting Free from Past or Present Pain) - Tapping with Brad Yates.* Narcissists (getting free from past or present pain) - Tapping with Brad Yates - YouTube

Zhang, M., Zhang, Y. & Kong, Y. (2020, May 18). *Interaction Between Social Pain and Physical Pain.* SAGE Journals. https://doi.org/10.26599%2FBSA.2019.9050023

Zwerican, A & Joseph, S. (2018, October 1). *Focusing Manner and Posttraumatic Growth.* Core. https://www.focusing.org.uk/an-introduction-to-focusing

YOUR FEEDBACK IS VALUED

From the bottom of our hearts, thank you for reading our book. We truly hope that it helps you on your spiritual journey and to live a more empowered and happy life. Would you be kind enough to leave an honest review for this book on Amazon? We would be ecstatic to hear your feedback. Thank you and good luck,

The Ascending Vibrations team

JOIN OUR COMMUNITY

Why not join our Facebook community and discuss your spiritual path with like-minded seekers?

We would love to hear from you.

Go to this link to join the 'Ascending Vibrations' community: bit.ly/ascendingvibrations

CLAIM YOUR FREE AUDIOBOOK

Download the 5+ Hour Audiobook *'Sound Healing For Beginners: Sonic Medicine Tor The Body, Chakra Rituals, & What They Didn't Tell You About Vibrational Energy'* Instantly for **FREE!**

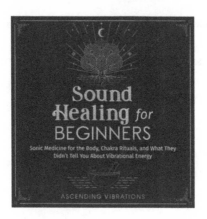

If you love listening to audio books on-the-go, we have great news for you. You can download the audio book version of *'Sound Healing For Beginners'* for **FREE** just by signing up for a **FREE** 30-day audible trial. See below for more details!

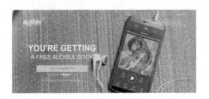

Audible trial benefits

As an audible customer, you'll receive the below benefits with your 30-day free trial:

- Free audible copy of this book
- After the trial, you will get 1 credit each month to use on any audiobook
- Your credits automatically roll over to the next month if you don't use them
- Choose from over 400,000 titles
- Listen anywhere with the audible app across multiple devices
- Make easy, no hassle exchanges of any audiobook you don't love
- Keep your audiobooks forever, even if you cancel your membership
- And much more

Click the links below to get started:
Go here for AUDIBLE US: adbl.co/3wk0Ahe
Go here for AUDIBLE UK: adbl.co/3stsPsV

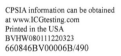